Crystal Healing for Women

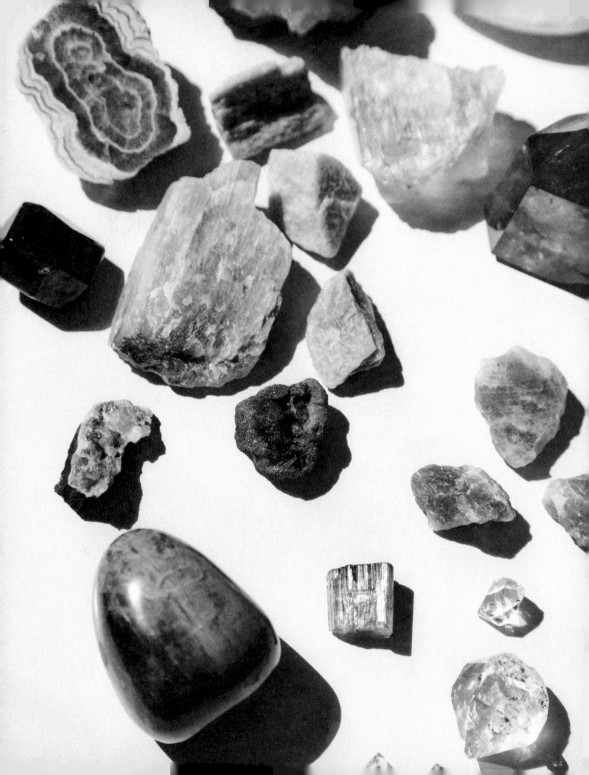

CRYSTAL HEALING
for WOMEN

A Modern Guide to the Power of Crystals for
Renewed Energy, Strength, and Wellness

Mariah K. Lyons

PHOTOGRAPHY BY AMY DICKERSON

ZEITGEIST • NEW YORK

Copyright © 2020 by Penguin Random House LLC

All rights reserved.

Published in the United States by Zeitgeist, an imprint of Zeitgeist™, a division of Penguin Random House LLC, New York.

penguinrandomhouse.com

Zeitgeist™ is a trademark of Penguin Random House LLC

ISBN: 9780593196823

Ebook ISBN: 9780593196830

Photography by Amy Dickerson

Illustration © Daryna Kurinna/Shutterstock.com (line art) and Mary Long/Shutterstock.com (chakra illustration)

Book design by Katy Brown

Printed in the United States of America

3 5 7 9 10 8 6 4 2

First Edition

To my mother, Maureen,
and to Mother Earth.

Contents

II
Energy, Strength, *and* Healing Rituals

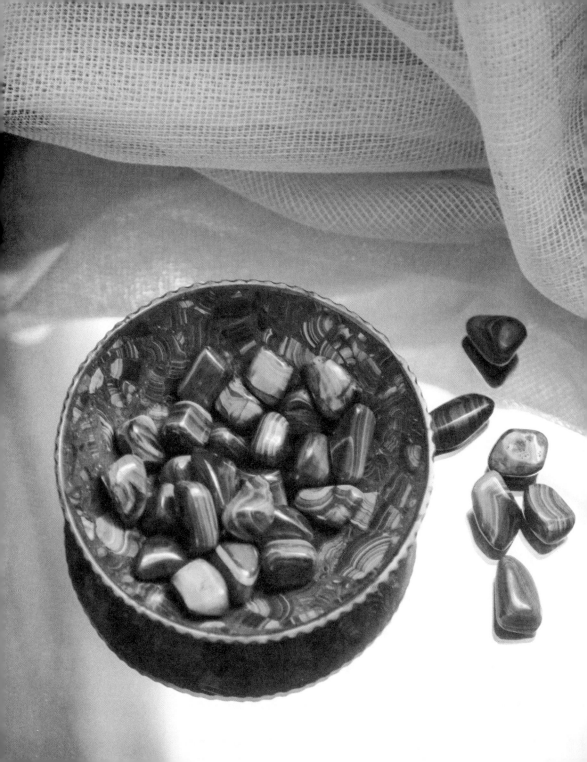

Introduction

IMAGINE A WORLD WHERE PEOPLE LIVE IN HARMONY WITH nature. Where they listen to her wisdom, live in tune with her cycle, honor each droplet of water, flower, and mineral—and where each step upon her belly is taken in prayer and reverence. Imagine a world where women fully awaken to the divinity and intuitive healing powers within themselves and where they remember their instinctual relationship with Mother Earth and the ancient wisdom she holds.

This is awakening now on our planet—and you are part of it! Your soul called you here, Earth called you here, and the crystals called you here. As the collective consciousness continues to shift on this planet, souls are waking up to their full potential. The crystals and the crystalline energy they anchor to this planet are here to support our evolution. In fact, many new powerful stones continue to be discovered every year, and these stones are exactly aligned with the energies we need as a collective at this stage in our journey. It is no coincidence that crystals have gained popularity in the last 50 years. This ancient form of healing, turned fringe modality, has made its way into all streams of life as we have now collectively reached a level of consciousness capable of implementing these high-frequency stones.

As we individually step into our true power and heal ourselves, we contribute to the healing of the planet. Healing within heals the world. We are on the precipice of great change, a time period in our evolution that has been written and prophesized in many ancient cultures. The world needs more awakened individuals and leaders in alignment with their truth and in deep connection with nature. We are the ones we've been waiting for! This book is intended to be a deep resource for accessing the codes held within the minerals that will help awaken you to your unlimited potential.

Along my path to healing, crystals have been my greatest allies. I'm deeply honored to share their medicine with you. Growing up in the mountains in Utah, I would often collect geodes and minerals from the mountains or desert with my father as well as different stones from the local trading posts. Being an imaginative and empathic child, I simply loved crystals. They felt magical, like a whole world was inside of them. While I had always had an innate, deep connection with animals and plants, speaking with them and communicating psychically as a child, it wasn't until young adulthood that the crystals began deeply communicating with me.

Crystals helped to awaken my own gifts and changed the course of my life along the way. From helping me heal autoimmune issues to manifesting incredible experiences in my life, the minerals have been a potent aspect of my journey every step of the way. In fact, many of the rituals in this book were rituals I channeled from the minerals to help myself heal and find well-being. In addition to helping me, the stones and rituals in this book also helped countless clients and community members to heal and fully awaken to the divine blueprint within themselves.

While this book is written as a comprehensive crystal healing book for women, it is intended to help heal and activate the feminine energy, regardless of gender identification. We do dive into the

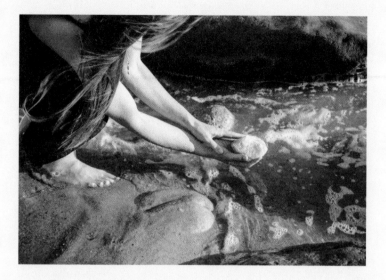

archetypal as well as biological cycles in a woman's life, but the information in this book can be applied to the feminine journey, regardless of how you identify (male, female, nonbinary, transgender, gender neutral, or any other identification).

It is my honor to guide you deeper into the mineral world so that you may intentionally utilize and incorporate crystals into your everyday life, helping you to find deeper levels of peace, self-love, joy, balance, and well-being. I invite you to stay neutral, curious, open-minded, and present as the magic unfolds. Crystals never "give" you anything you don't already have—they help you to uncover what has been there all along. They are extremely powerful tools of transformation, healing, and creation and are to be honored as such. We are here to heal individually and collectively, creating the new world we wish to see. Enjoy your journey into the world of mineral healing, unlocking the magic available to us every day.

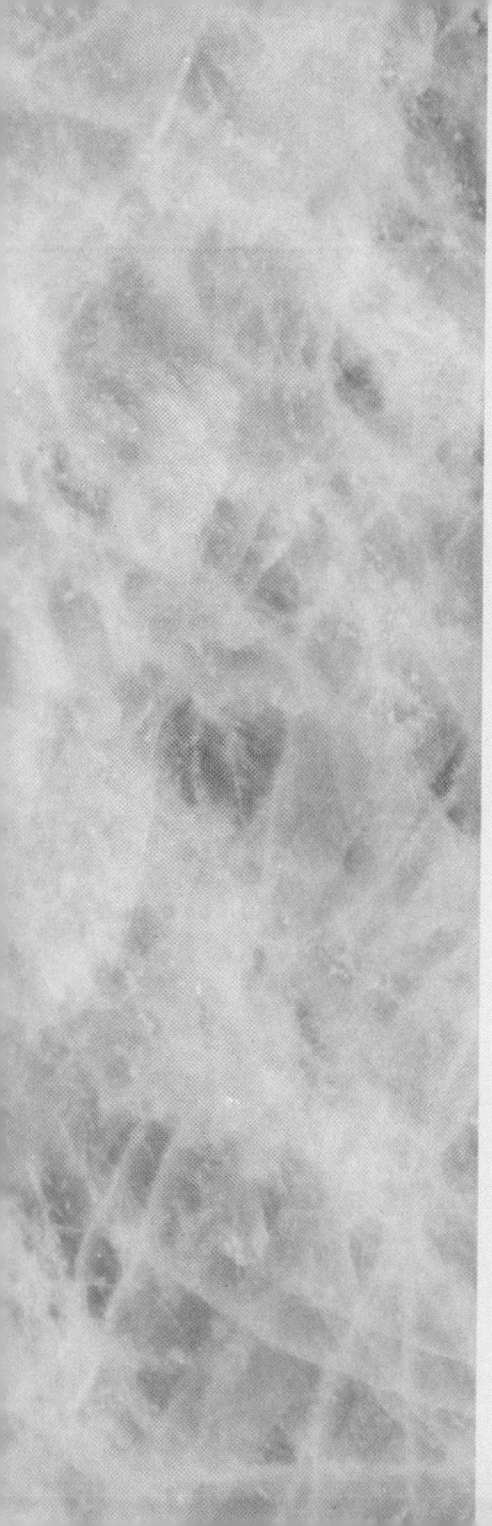

*
*
*

I

THE
HEALING
POWER
of
CRYSTALS

*
*
*

If you want to find the secrets

of the universe, you must

think in terms of energy,

frequency, and vibration.

—NIKOLA TESLA

ONE

Unlocking Crystal Energy

CRYSTALS HELP TO UNLOCK MANY ANCIENT SECRETS OF healing and the wisdom held within the earth. But how can a rock you found online do that? It all has to do with frequency and vibration. Crystals are the original thumb drives. They are often called the "wisdom keepers of Earth," as they literally store information in the form of vibration within their molecular structure. They have much information to share with us, information that has been held within the earth for millions of years. We are being called now to unlock these mysteries so that we may shift the energy of the planet toward that of harmony and union, not only for ourselves but also for the collective.

What Are Crystals?

Well, you're made of them! Your teeth and bones are composed of an aragonite and calcite crystalline structure, and the microscopic calcite crystals in your ear help you maintain your balance. And without even knowing it, minerals are already a key component in your everyday life! From table salt (halite), to pencil lead (graphite), to your cell phone (quartz crystals), to wristwatches (quartz crystals), minerals are an integral part of life on Earth.

There are over 4,000 different types of minerals currently found on the planet—and new discoveries are made each year! Nowadays, we often hear the words *crystals, minerals, gems, stones,* and *rocks* used interchangeably, but what exactly is a crystal? Geologists define crystal as a solid substance with an organized structure and repeating geometric pattern, known as a *crystal lattice.* Crystallization occurs as a result of temperature changes or pressure. Crystals can be naturally occurring or artificially made. For example, water molecules become crystallized by freezing, and diamonds are formed by intense pressure and heat. For the purposes of this book, we recognize that healing crystals may also be minerals, rocks, or gemstones with useful energetic properties.

Crystal Energy and Vibration

Everything in this universe vibrates at a particular frequency. What your eye sees as physical, solid matter is in fact vibrating particles of matter condensed and slowed into form. Einstein's famous equation $E = mc^2$ reflects this, saying that everything is both vibration *and* matter. Matter is simply vibrating energy that is slow enough for our senses to perceive.

This energy creates a naturally occurring electromagnetic field. You, too, have an electromagnetic field, also called an *energetic field* or *auric field*. It is the energy field around your body (or any living thing) created by electrical currents within the body. The heart produces the highest electrical current within the body, even higher than the waves created by the brain. Your energy field varies in strength, magnetism, and radiance, depending upon your emotional, mental, and physical well-being.

Vibrational frequencies vary in tone, from high to low. An example of these gradations in frequency can be found in color and sound waves. On a color spectrum, violet is a very fast frequency of light, while red is slower and denser. In music, notes vibrate at different levels, and our ears register these sounds as higher- or lower-pitched frequency tones. Sound waves and light frequencies are energetic vibrations that can be seen and felt.

Crystals vibrate energy in the exact same way. They each have a particular tonality or frequency that radiates from within the crystal lattice structure. Some crystals have a higher or finer vibration, while other stones resonate at a slower or denser frequency. Neither is better nor worse, just as red and violet are neither better nor worse colors; they are simply different.

With crystal energy, we use the frequency at which the crystal resonates to harmonize and heal imbalances within our energetic field on a quantum and cellular level. For example, when you feel anxious or have had too many cups of coffee in one sitting, the energetic level in your body often increases and your heart begins vibrating at a rapid pace. Working with a high-frequency crystal would exacerbate these sensations. Instead, reaching for a stone that is grounding and has a slower vibration would bring you back into the body and present moment.

As your body vibrates energy, it can align with the frequencies of the stone to harmonize energetic levels within your body's electromagnetic field. When the energy within your body is in balance and in flow, there is health and well-being in many areas of life. However, when energy is blocked, illness, disease, and imbalances can occur. This blocked flow can occur as a result of past or present trauma, stress, fear, stored/unprocessed/suppressed emotions, bodily injuries, and scar tissue, as well as collective or ancestral patterning still present in your DNA.

Think of the natural energetic flow in your body as a river. If something impedes the water and prevents it from flowing, it will begin to pool, and that fresh flow of water will eventually become a stagnant swamp. When blockage or stagnation happens with the river of life force within your body, illness and energetic imbalance occur. By allowing your natural life

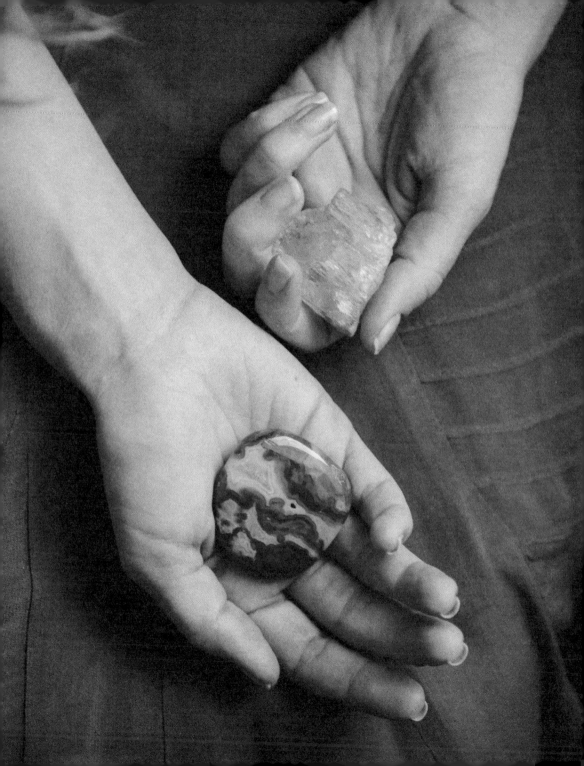

DIVINE FEMININE ENERGY

The Divine Feminine energy is reawakening on our planet. It is an energy that exists within all of us, regardless of gender identification, but has been suppressed for hundreds of years by the dominant and out-of-balance masculine energy. This has not always been the case. There was a time in ancient cultures when humans were in conscious relationship with Mother Nature and the Divine Feminine—a time when this energy was deeply honored, revered, and respected as the energies of the Great Mother and the Goddess. As the Divine Feminine energy is once again rising on the planet, we are coming back into balance and harmony with Mother Nature and the feminine energies within ourselves.

Feminine energy is seen as yin, cold, dark, receptive, creative, right-brain, subconscious, and nonlinear, while masculine is yang, hot, light, active, analytical, left-brain, conscious and linear. When we are balanced in our masculine and feminine energies, the information and creative insight we receive in the feminine connect with the masculine energy of action and structure, and we are then able to translate creative visions into the physical world. It is a harmonizing, energetic partnership.

The Divine Feminine is quantum. She is in everything. She is soft, nurturing, graceful, intuitive, gentle, wise, deeply empathic, and sensitive. She is also strong, fierce, determined, courageous, wild, untamed, passionate, juicy, and life-giving; yet simultaneously holds death, destruction, decay, and then rebirth. The Divine Feminine is all encompassing. She is not only within you—she is you.

The rituals and practices in this book will help you attune to the energies of Mother Nature as well as harness, heal, and awaken the Divine Feminine energy within.

force to flow fluidly, your body can restore itself to its natural state of harmony and balance, where it can utilize and direct vital prana (or life-force energy) to experience high levels of energy, function, and well-being. You are naturally radiant! It is your natural state of being. Your healing journey simply requires removing whatever is blocking your natural state of flow and realigning to your divine state of innate perfection.

Crystal Healing in History

For millennia, the use of minerals and gemstones has proved to be an integral aspect of holistic well-being in healing and has been found in cultures all over the world, including the Aztecs and Incas, Indian sages, Native Americans, the Maori, the Celts, the ancient Greeks, and the ancient Egyptians.

Ayurvedic healers and astrologers in India and Tibet have considered gemstones and crystals to be important elements in aligning one's overall vitality and counterbalancing planetary influences based on individual astrology for thousands of years. Gemstones are prescribed to individuals and placed on specific areas of the body to harmonize and heal imbalances based on that person's Ayurvedic constitution and their Vedic astrology.

Ancient Egyptians heavily adorned their temples, jewelry, and burial sarcophagi with minerals of the local region. Crystals were used in ceremonial rituals and ancient healing practices, and powdered stones were used for colored pigment for art and makeup. It is believed that Cleopatra's iconic cat-eye eyeshadow and eyeliner were made from finely ground lapis lazuli and malachite and that she wore it both for beauty and to support seeing beyond the visible reality.

In ancient China, emperors and military leaders were buried in full bodysuits made of jade. Jade has been mined, traded, and highly revered in China for 11,000 years. Confucius even wrote in the *Book of Odes*, "When I think of a wise man, his merits appear to be like Jade."

The direct application of crystalline energy is seen not only in ancient and modern healing, but also in much of our modern-day technology, which either utilizes the energy of crystals or is based off the scientific principle of piezoelectricity found in crystals. Piezoelectricity was discovered in 1880 by French scientists Paul-Jacques Curie and Pierre Curie, when they found that mechanically pressurizing certain crystals created an electric charge. This form of electricity is now found everywhere in many modern applications, including radio transmissions, cell phones, wristwatches, microphones, earbuds, televisions, and computer motherboards. There's even a subway station is Japan that utilizes the piezoelectric pressure caused by the weight of the commuters in front of turnstiles to create electricity that powers its power ticket gates and electronic displays.

While the modern applications of crystals are vast, science is just beginning to scratch the surface of the information and power stored for thousands (oftentimes millions) of years within Earth's crystals.

The Role of Color in Healing

As we are sensory beings, our senses—even our eyes—can help us heal. Chromotherapy is one such form of healing that utilizes the visible waves of electromagnetic radiation, or what our eyes register as color, to treat various ailments. A modern form of chromotherapy is light therapy that uses blue, red, and white light to treat various ailments, including depression, acne, and neurological disorders. It stimulates stem cell regeneration and wound healing. The art of healing with color and light has a long-standing history; records of color healing dating back to 2000 BC have been found in ancient Egypt, Greece, India, and China. In fact, not only were gemstones, colored garments, and colored salves and ointments used, but also temples and healing rooms were often painted certain colors to elicit additional healing and balancing qualities.

The additional mineral components within crystals can amplify the healing qualities of color in a variety of ways:

WHITE is a reflective and protective color and contains all the colors on the light spectrum. This high-frequency color aids in detoxification and bringing one's energy inward and is therefore an ideal color to wear when you're meditating, feeling unwell, or in need of a radiance boost.

YELLOW AND GOLD are activating, energizing, and joy-enhancing colors. They can stimulate cognitive functioning and support the nervous and digestive systems. They boost self-confidence and courage, and it can help lift depressive moods.

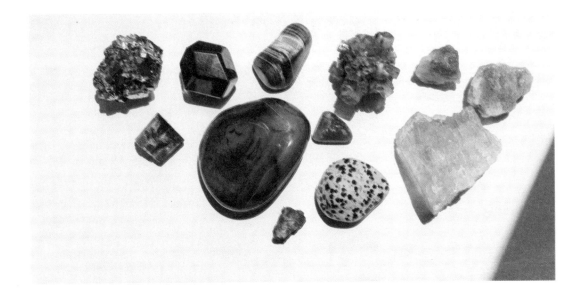

ORANGE is a warm, creative, sensual, and invigorating color. It can help boost the immune system, stimulate the thyroid, increase circulation, and activate sexual energy.

BROWN is grounding and nourishing to the system. It creates a sense of safety and security.

PINK is the color of unconditional love. It opens the heart to compassion and forgiveness of others and can soothe anxiety, fear, and sadness. It is also an extremely protective color. A color of self-defense, it harmonizes energies around it and neutralizes negative energies.

RED is the color of passion, security, and sexuality. It ignites the flame within, creating a warming and activating sensation. It can help increase circulation, support menstruation and ovulation, and stimulate your sex drive.

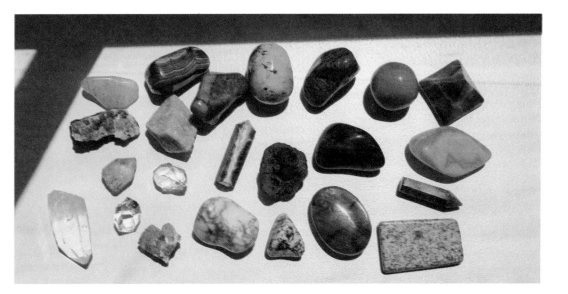

PURPLE AND VIOLET are colors of transformation and release. They help with insomnia, addictive behavior, and negative thinking patterns, and can help relieve pain and bring a sense of peace and calm to the mind.

BLUE is one of the most healing, soothing colors on the spectrum and helps bring the mind into a meditative state. It aids in calming the nervous system and lowering inflammation within the body.

GREEN is the color of love, nature, and natural divine abundance. It aids in healing the lungs and blockages related to heartbreak or grief. Green is a wonderful color for healing and bringing balance to the mental, emotional, and physical body.

GRAY is a neutral color and can allow for release, detoxification, and cleansing of your energy field. It is calming and allows you to stay neutral and impartial and decide how you wish to proceed.

BLACK is the color of mystery and of the void. It is a wonderful color for deep meditation and when tuning into the unknown. It can create a grounding and protective feeling.

Working with certain colors in crystals, herbs, and clothing can help balance your energy centers. Color healing also comes into play when balancing your seven main chakra centers (page 57); each center corresponds with and vibrates to a particular color frequency.

Think about your closet and how you feel throughout the day when you wear certain colors. I tend to wear a lot of neutral colors like white, blush, gray, and black, as they are grounding and help me stay in a space of openness and neutrality when working. However, I love to activate and channel different energies by wearing vibrant jewel-toned colors for special occasions—I might throw on red heels for a date night with my husband, a yellow blouse for a speaking event, or pink for a wedding. Think about your own clothing: What colors excite you and help you feel expansive and creative when you wear them? Which ones feel grounding and protective?

THE ROLE OF RITUALS IN HEALING

A ritual practice can be deeply nourishing and grounding along your spiritual journey. The practice of ritual combines sacred intention with action. Rituals help bridge the realms of the mystical with the material and can serve as powerful portals to healing and conscious creation. Engaging in daily, weekly, monthly, or seasonal rituals can help you to stay present in your daily life and along your unique soul's journey.

Certain rituals presented in this book are exceptionally potent during certain times of the day, month, or year. This is because the practice of aligning with the cosmic cycles of Earth, planets, and stars helps you attune to the rhythms of nature. The amplified energies available for healing and quantum manifestation during celestial activations can also supercharge your rituals. The rituals included in this book help you bring alignment, healing, and well-being into your life.

A daily ritual practice is an incredible grounding tool for deep healing and transformation. Whether it be a daily meditation practice, personal crystal healing, sacred movement, or a nightly bath ritual, a daily dedicated ritual practice is one of the most potent tools for integrated healing.

Look deep into nature, and then you

will understand everything better.

—ALBERT EINSTEIN

TWO

Collecting and Caring for Crystals

ARE YOU READY TO UNCOVER THE HEALING POTENTIAL of minerals? This chapter explores the intuitive process of crystal selection, as well as cleansing and programming. Look upon each step of the process as a way to strengthen the intuition and guidance found within you as you select stones based on vibrational alignment, cleanse with the elements of Earth, and come into deep relationship with your new crystal allies. As you become a crystals caretaker, you'll have the responsibility of caring for Earth, stewarding the wisdom and healing potential of the mineral world, and discovering the powerful healer within you.

Buying Crystals

If you are at the beginning of your crystal healing journey, I recommend starting with just one to three crystals (see Chapters 4 and 5 for crystal options). Get to know their energetic qualities, and grow your relationship with them for a few months before adding more. This way you will deeply understand the profiles and frequencies of the minerals, and they can become deep allies and healing tools for the future.

When buying crystals, pay close attention to how you feel when you first hold or see (especially if buying online) a crystal. Look for the initial feeling of connection, attraction, or expansion within you. Try to energetically attune with the crystal first—before reading its description. Usually, the healing crystal that you are originally drawn to will be a perfect match for what your body and spirit need at that time. If you select stones based on their description, your mind or ego may make the selection rather than your intuition.

It can be difficult to determine the fair price of a particular crystal because crystal prices range widely. This is due to the various factors involved, including the rarity of the gem, the quality of the mineral, and its cut, size, and location of origin. If you are buying a larger or rare specimen, it is always a good idea to first cross-check prices online or with other dealers.

Earth-Made or Laboratory-Made Crystals

In recent years, as demand for crystals has increased and supply for certain stones has decreased, there has been an influx of laboratory-made and altered crystals. While laboratory-manufactured crystals do contain healing qualities relating to their respective color, they don't possess the energy and information from the earth. I personally prefer natural, untreated crystals, meaning stones that are not heated or dyed to achieve a specific color, as they hold the original informational intent and healing qualities of the earth. However, it is all up to you. Always trust your intuition!

Polished or Organic Crystals

There is a slight energetic difference between a natural raw stone and a polished, tumbled, or cut stone. A natural stone is in its original form, while the cut or polished stone has undergone an additional process to resize or smooth it. However,

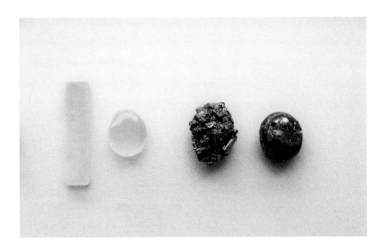

23

the difference is so slight that it's not worth worrying over; instead, think about how comfortable it feels. For some, it can be distracting to place a raw-edged stone against their skin during a ritual or meditation. If that is the case for you, a smooth tumbled stone that fits perfectly in your hand may be more relaxing to the senses and help you move into deeper states of healing. It ultimately comes down to personal preference.

Where to Buy

You can buy crystals from physical stores, online boutiques, mineral shows, and even Amazon! When first working with crystals, it is a good idea to see and feel them in person, either in a physical store or at a gem and mineral show. Mineral shows offer an opportunity to see and feel a variety of stones. The biggest gem and mineral shows in the world take place every winter in Tucson, but you can find local mineral shows in every state throughout the year.

Crystals hold on to frequency and energetic information, which means they absorb the energetic imprint of how they were mined, the person distributing them, the shipping facilitators, and so on. You will have a cleaner and higher vibrational stone when it is honored every step of the way. With practice, you can feel the difference between a stone that was mined and sold with integrity and reverence and one that was mined in the energy of greed and environmental negligence.

When shopping for crystals online, find a reputable dealer. I've found that stones purchased from small, thoughtfully curated shops tend to have higher-quality crystals than large retailers. You might pay a bit more, but it is worth it in the long run. Again, quality and integrity first and foremost.

Identifying Crystal Shapes

While the intrinsic qualities of a stone are not altered when it is cut or polished, the overall shape of the crystal does affect the flow of energy. How you intend to use the crystal will help determine which shape (raw or sculpted) you should choose.

SINGLE CRYSTAL POINT: A crystal point is a single terminated crystal and is great for directing energy. It acts like an arrow, focusing energy and intention in one specific direction. You may use a crystal point for manifestation, self-healing, and crystal grid work.

WAND: The crystal wand shape helps to direct the energy of a stone in a particular direction. It may be natural in shape, such as a selenite wand, or cut and polished to achieve the desired shape, such as in a massage wand or a double terminated wand. Wands are great for placing on the body as well as in crystal grids because they greatly facilitate energy flow.

DOUBLE TERMINATED CRYSTAL: A double terminated crystal is a single crystal with a point at each end. It both sends and receives energy simultaneously, moving energy quickly and clearing stagnation. A double termination cleanses old energy as it brings in a fresh vibrant flow, making it a great fit for personal energy balancing. Try placing it on your womb after menstruation to fully release energetic residue from the previous month and welcome in the energy of a new cycle.

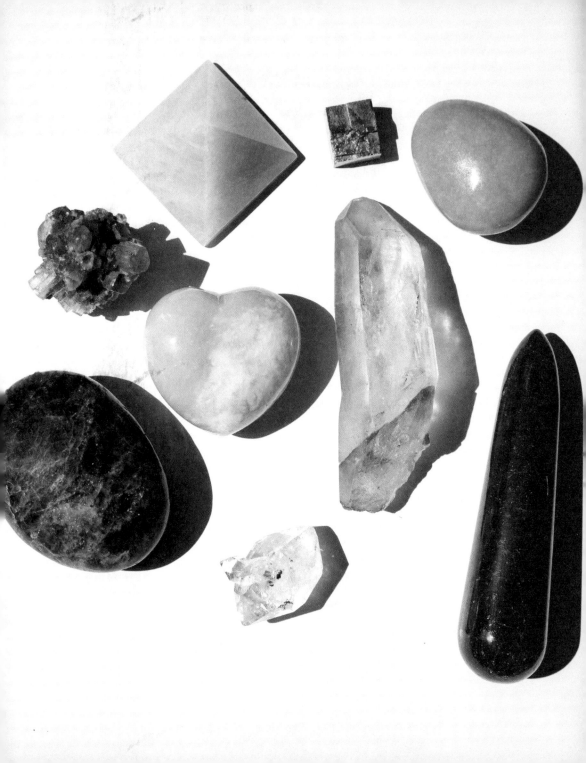

CLUSTER: A cluster is a group or family of crystal points that grow from the same unified base. A crystal cluster can bring the energy of unity and togetherness into an environment. It's wonderful for bringing harmony and cohesiveness to group dynamics among families, offices, community spaces, group meditations, and so on.

TUMBLED/PALM STONES: Tumbled stones and palm stones are polished and tumbled to achieve a smooth surface. Their shape makes them conducive to meditation, bath rituals, self-healing, and carrying with you while out and about.

HEART: A polished heart crystal is cut and polished into the shape of a heart. It works with the Heart Chakra and helps you attune to the energy of universal love. It can be a powerful shape to work with in meditation and healing, particularly in self-love practices and rituals for attracting new love.

PYRAMID: The pyramid shape enhances the channeling of specific energy. It is a potent crystal shape to work with in crystal grids and manifestation practices because it creates a vortex of energy lifting up toward the cosmos, bridging earth and sky while bringing intentions and prayers into the ethers.

SPHERE: A sphere shape is complete, whole in itself and doesn't contain any hard or cornered edges. It helps to radiate crystalline energy in all directions. A sphere is a wonderful crystal shape to have in your home and place of work. It also connects to radiant circular energy of the Divine Feminine.

EGG: An egg is one of the most ancient symbols of the Divine Feminine. In certain cultures, the Universe is said to have been born from a golden egg-shaped womb. Egg-shaped crystals connect to the eternal creative energy within us all and are often found in crystal yoni eggs. Crystal eggs are a potent shape to work with for creativity rituals, fertility practices, and conscious conception.

CUBE: A cube maintains powerful structure and is the foundational geometric shape of building. It anchors energy into a particular area and is a potent shape for grounding and rooting. A cube crystal connects to the energy of the Divine Masculine. Use it when you need to bring more structure into your life or ground the energy of the room, such as rooms with Wi-Fi routers.

Getting to Know Your Crystals

You've chosen your first crystals . . . now what? When initially getting to know a crystal and how it uniquely attunes to your energy, stay open, curious, and playful. You may introduce yourself to your crystal if you wish, as it is a new ally and friend you are bringing into your life. One of the first stones I truly fell in love with and became a student of was a labradorite. I carried him everywhere and meditated deeply with him for over a year (I say *him* because the energy of the stone presented masculine to me). The more I meditated with the healing crystal and stayed open to the information that came through, the more I trusted him as an ally and the more I opened up to more layers within myself. So, allow your relationship with your crystal to ripen over time.

Everyone feels and experiences crystals differently, just as everyone has their own unique gifts and ways of interpreting information from the Universe. Some people feel physical sensations within their body when holding crystals, others might receive visuals or hear words, while others may simply feel calm and an overall sense of grounding. Your experience with crystals will continue to shift over time, so stay open and in a state of wonder and awe as you experience the beauty of yourself through the stones.

At first, simply notice how you feel when looking at the crystal or holding it. What does it evoke in you? What feeling or image comes forth that you wish to explore? Again, there is nothing within the crystal that you don't have within you. It's a keycode, so to speak, to access deeper layers within your energetic coding and soul lineage through a process of self-exploration and self-healing. Here are some initial steps to help you engage your crystal:

1   Hold the stone in your hand and close your eyes.

2   Take a few deep breaths and envision the crystal's energy gently melding into your body and energy field.

3   Feel your body begin to adjust to this new tone. Notice any subtle shifts within your body or sensations that arise. Perhaps you hear a word/phrase or a memory/image comes

to mind. Stay open, neutral, and present with any and all shifts that occur.

4   Pay attention to how you feel after holding the crystal.

5   Write down any notes, insights, visions, or feelings that came forth.

Each crystal is special, and the more you tune into it, the more your relationship will deepen. Just like any relationship, the more you honor, respect, and intentionally work with your crystal, the more you will benefit from it in your life. As the crystal is now officially in your care, it is time to attune the stone to your energy field by cleansing, clearing, and programming your stone to your specific intentions!

Cleansing Your Crystals

Imagine unknowingly buying a hard drive that was already filled up with data. In order to save any new information to it, you'd need to delete the previous owner's files first. This is what happens when we cleanse our crystals; it is the energetic version of CTR-ALT-DELETE. Crystals not only store the energy of Earth, but they also absorb the energy of their caretakers and environments. As you can imagine, they can get quite filled up! Sometimes this can be physically seen, such as in a clear quartz that becomes milky or cloudy over time.

It is important to cleanse your crystals when you first receive them and periodically afterward, depending upon usage. For healing rituals, it is important to cleanse the stones both before and after use. This ensures the stone is vibrating at a pure frequency before your ritual, and any heavy energy released during the healing is cleansed from the crystal afterward. This is an important part of what I call "crystal energetic hygienics."

The more you work with your crystals, the more you will tune into the subtle changes that signify when it is time to cleanse them. They may look murky or take on a slightly heavy and dense feel. They might not have as strong or potent a vibration as they once did, almost like a weak or faint pulse. If it is a stone you wear constantly, such as a wedding ring, necklace, or earrings, you might notice feelings of agitation, anxiety, anger, or fear. This is because these stones are consistently exposed to many different environments, people, and energies, and they can absorb a great deal of these external frequencies as well as your own. Don't panic and feel you need to energetically cleanse your jewelry all the time—just stay aware of how they are vibrationally radiating. I always make sure to cleanse my jewelry after long trips, being in airports or large crowds, or during periods of great change and transformation in my own life, as I know these stones are helping me to facilitate these changes and help restore balance.

Water Cleansing

Water is a beautiful tool for cleansing your crystals. The element of water helps to release and move stored energy within the stones. Not all stones are compatible with water, though, so please reference the crystal profiles in Chapters Four and Five. Here are some different ways to cleanse with water:

- Place your stones under running water, such as a faucet or shower, for 30 seconds.
- Place your stones in a white ceramic or glass container with a pinch of sea salt. Let sit for 10 to 30 minutes.
- Rinse your stones in the ocean or hold them under the current of a river, stream, or creek. Be careful not to lose the stones in the current.

Sacred Herbs and Smoke

Many ancient traditions incorporate the use of burning sacred herbs and resins for clearing stagnant and heavy energy. Light the herb, incense, or resin and allow the smoke to billow around the crystal for 10 to 30 seconds. Watch the smoke envelop the stone and set the intention for cleansing. Here are some herbs and resins that are often used for this purpose:

- White sage
- Palo Santo
- Rosemary
- Cinnamon stick
- Copal
- Incense
- Cedar
- Juniper
- Frankincense

Sound Currents

The wavelengths from particular sounds can also loosen energy from the stones and help to cleanse them. As with all cleansing practices, set the intention for cleansing before playing the instruments. Let the sound currents fully bathe the crystals for 1 to 5 minutes.

Consider using any of these instruments or tools for cleansing:

* Chime
* Drum
* Tuning fork
* Crystal singing bowl

Cleansing with Rice

White rice is highly absorbent and will help to soak up any dense or heavy energy from your stones. Quickly cleanse with water (only when applicable) beforehand, and then simply place your crystals in a bowl of white rice overnight. Throw the rice out onto the earth in the morning so it can transform the energy; a garden, compost pile, or under a tree are nice regenerative spots.

Crystals as Cleansers

A few crystals act as cleansers and chargers for other crystals. Selenite, kyanite, and moldavite can both cleanse and charge other minerals. Place the stone being cleansed on top of the cleansing stone and maintain direct contact for 30 minutes to 1 hour.

Cleansing with the Earth

Another way to completely restore the energy of a stone is to bury it in the earth. The earth will absorb any stagnant energy from the stone and restore it back into balance with the frequency of the earth. Bury it on the full moon and keep it there until the next full moon. Just don't forget where you buried it!

CRYSTAL GIFTS

When selecting a crystal for another person as a gift, the first step is to tune into the energy of the recipient. Close your eyes, say the person's name in your mind, and visualize them standing in front of you. Then ask yourself what energy would be supportive for them. Stay open to any words, colors, images, and feelings that arise, and then select the crystal based on that.

BIRTHSTONES

Birthstones correlate to the energies of the months and can be beautiful in jewelry or hand stones.

January: Garnet
February: Amethyst
March: Aquamarine
April: Diamond
May: Emerald
June: Pearl and moonstone
July: Ruby
August: Peridot
September: Sapphire
October: Opal and tourmaline
November: Citrine and topaz
December: Turquoise

BIRTHDAYS

Celebrate a solar return (aka birthday) with crystals that bring energetic blessings of love, abundance, prosperity, and good health.

* Citrine
* Clear quartz
* Jade
* Peridot
* Rose quartz
* Ruby

BRIDAL SHOWERS

These stones connect to the Divine Feminine energy and celebrate a new phase in a woman's life:

* Angelite
* Blue-lace agate
* Kunzite
* Moonstone
* Pearl
* Ruby

WEDDINGS

These stones enhance the energies of deep soul love, divine partnership, prosperity, and good health:

* Aventurine
* Citrine
* Jade
* Peridot
* Rose quartz
* Turquoise
* Twin clear quartz points

GRADUATION

These stones are beautiful gifts that invoke the energies of focus, self-reliance, courage, creativity, protection, and good luck:

* Blue apatite
* Blue kyanite
* Citrine
* Clear quartz
* Iolite
* Jade
* Peridot
* Pyrite
* Smoky quartz

HOUSEWARMING

Offer these stones to help create a peaceful, warm, inviting, safe, grounded, and love-filled space:

* Amethyst
* Apophyllite
* Black onyx
* Celestite
* Jade
* Petrified wood
* Rose quartz
* Ruby
* Selenite

NEW BABY

These stones emanate peaceful, loving, healing, and pure vibrations for a nursery or child's room:

* Angelite
* Apophyllite
* Calcite
* Celestite
* Jade
* Lemurian seed
* Lepidolite
* Peach moonstone
* Rose quartz
* Scolecite

NEW JOB/PROMOTION

These crystals radiate energies of courage, strength, protection, and prosperity:

* Aragonite
* Citrine
* Hematite
* Peridot
* Pyrite
* Selenite

Charging Your Crystals

In addition to cleansing, charging your crystals is part of your crystal energetic hygiene—but they're different processes. Think of cleansing as taking a bath or shower to release residue, and think of charging as eating nutritious foods that bring your energy levels up. Charging helps to strengthen and maintain the vibration of your gemstone and can boost certain tones and frequencies within the crystal.

Contrary to popular belief, when you place your stones in the moonlight or sunlight, you are actually charging them with lunar and solar energy, not cleansing them. You can also charge stones with certain frequencies of power places throughout the world, such as Glastonbury, Mt. Shasta, Hawaii, Lake Titicaca, or your favorite places in nature.

Sunbath or Solar Charging

A sunbath provides a more masculine charge to crystals. It's great for stones with a Divine Masculine energy, like malachite and tiger's eye, and stones that you are working with in manifestation practices. Place your stones in the sunlight (the best hours are between sunrise and 11:00 A.M. or between 4:00 P.M. and sundown) for at least 10 minutes but no more than 2 hours. Sunlight can damage certain stones, so it's best not to place them in high midday heat or for extended periods of time. The spring equinox and summer solstice are great days for solar charging.

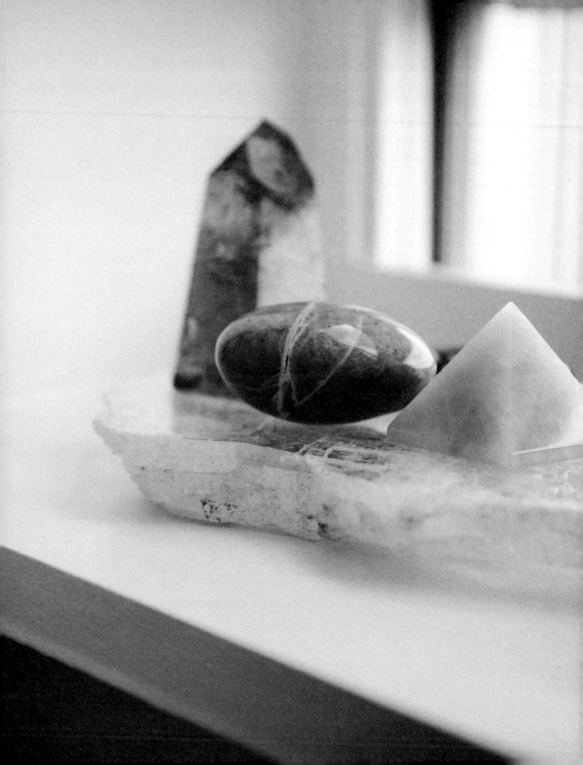

Moonbath or Lunar Charging

The moon heightens the feminine aspects of a crystal, so moonbaths are great for boosting the feminine energies of stones before fertility rituals and conception. It is also a good method for charging stones, like moonstone, ruby, amethyst, and lapis lazuli, which can boost intuition and creativity.

Begin by placing your crystals in a safe place outside in the light of the full moon. It's best to do this on the full moon, but it can be done within 48 hours of the full moon. Place the crystals ideally on a white towel or in a white ceramic or glass container, as it attracts the full light of the moon and does not interfere with any frequencies coming from colors (e.g., from a colorful towel).

If you're looking for a balanced feminine and masculine charge, place stones in the light of the full moon overnight, then leave in the sun for up to 2 hours in the morning. This will give the stones a lunar-solar boost. This is my favorite method for fully supercharged and balanced crystals!

Place of Power Charging

Take your stones to a personal place of power for you, perhaps a favorite place in nature or somewhere else that feels empowering to you. Leave your crystals on the ground to soak in the energy, and set the intention that this energy is stored within the crystal. Your stones can activate the place of power and bring its energy to you in other environments, such as your home.

TRUSTING YOUR INTUITION

Intuition is a beautiful gift we were all given at birth to help us navigate our lives in true alignment with our souls. It is not something some people have access to and others don't; we are all naturally intuitive beings! Our intuition helps us decipher the messages of our hearts and differentiate that which comes from the mind or from societal expectations. Sometimes our intuition comes as a whisper; other times it may shout. Over time, we begin to truly learn to trust our intuition above everything else. We strengthen our intuition by listening and then acting in accordance with that guidance. Then we repeat that process over and over again until our intuition becomes our true navigational system, an internal compass we can use every step along our winding journey.

When beginning to reestablish and trust your deep intuition, take time to get quiet. Ask yourself questions, stay neutral to the response you receive, and listen to the guidance that wells forth from within. Then take action on that guidance, even the small internal nudges. This is how you build and strengthen your lifelong relationship with your powerful intuition.

Crystal to Crystal Charging

Selenite, kyanite, and moldavite are all self-cleansing, high-frequency stones, meaning they vibrate at such a rapid pace that they cleanse and charge themselves. These stones can also help charge your other crystals. Simply place your crystal on top of selenite, kyanite, or moldavite and let sit for 30 minutes to 24 hours. I love this method for charging stones on delicate jewelry because it's convenient and safe.

Programming Your Crystals

An honest and pure intention is key in programming your crystals and achieving your desired results. Truly, the simpler the better. Once you are clear on your intention, simply hold the stone in your hand, close your eyes, and connect to your heart. Connect to the energy of the stone, and visualize your intention coming to full fruition. Now state your intention aloud or in your mind, and imagine the vibrations of the words you speak imprinting within the coding of the crystal. You are writing a clear code of what you want it to activate and radiate into the quantum field. Feel your heart expand with gratitude—you might even say "thank you" to the stone.

The crystal will hold the vibration of what you want to create and help reorganize the energy within your energetic field to support manifestation. However, you will need to take action, maintain clear vision, and practice unconditional trust in the Universe as you continue to work with your crystal. These are the magical keys that unlock the unlimited potential of crystal healing.

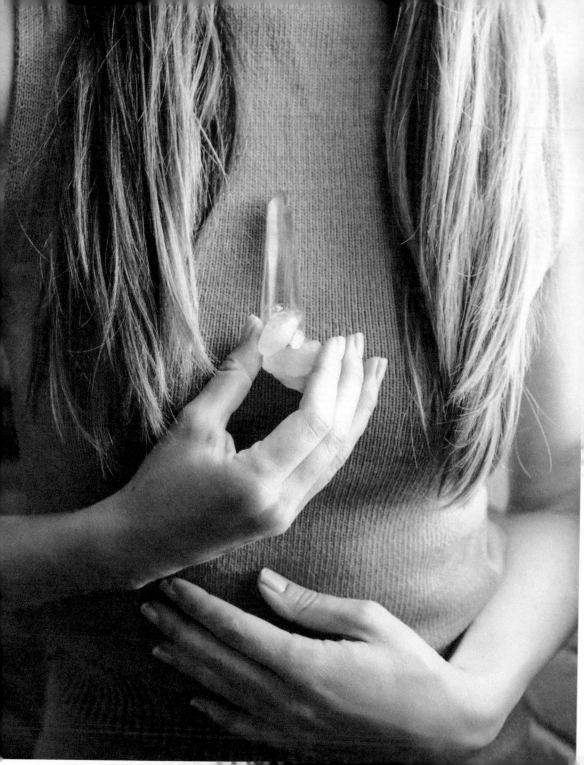

When women take care of

their health, they become

their own best friend.

—MAYA ANGELOU

THREE

Engaging Your Crystals

N OW THAT YOU HAVE CLEANSED AND PROGRAMMED your crystals, it is time to put them into action. Crystals love to be interacted with, not simply placed on a shelf and forgotten about. There is an energy exchange that happens when you engage with your stones that helps to further activate the stone and strengthen your connection to it. The more you intentionally work with your crystals and develop an understanding of how they interact with you, as well as the energy around them, the deeper your relationship will become and the more you will receive from the stone!

Clearing and Cleansing Your Space

Our physical environment often reflects our internal land-scape. I can tell in my own life that I'm overextending myself or not creating enough time for my grounding self-care practices when piles of laundry begin to stack up and my house becomes cluttered. When this happens, I will clear my schedule as best I can, turn off my phone, clean the house, energetically cleanse my space with herbs or resins, rearrange my crystals, and display fresh flowers. It instantly releases stagnant and dense energy and elevates the vibration of the house to a higher frequency, helping to anchor me back into my center and place of power within.

Cleansing and clearing the energy of your space alchemi-cally shifts the overall frequency of your home, helping to restore balance and bring deeper levels of healing into your life. Just as practices such as meditation, movement, rituals, energy healing, and working with sacred plants and minerals can help to cleanse your mind, body, and spirit, there are many ways you can energetically cleanse your physical spaces for overall well-being. Healing music, such as music at 528 Hz or 432 Hz; sacred mantras; and chanting music can also help to cleanse and elevate the space of your home.

Many of the same tools you use to cleanse your crystals, like herbs, plants, and resins, may also be used to cleanse your home. When working with these sacred tools, it is impor-tant to honor their place of origin and distribution. In recent years, plants such as white sage and Palo Santo have become

CLEANSING WITH SACRED SMOKE

The ancient practice of transforming energy through the use of burning sacred herbs, resins, and incense attunes the individual to the wisdom, power, and healing available through a conscious relationship with the plant. It also allows the smoke of the plant to cleanse and release energy from the body, an object, or the environment. From the burning of myrrh resin in ancient Egypt to the burning of white sage in many nations of the indigenous peoples of the Americas, including the Navajo and the Ute tribes, the ceremonial ritual burning of certain sacred herbs has a deep-seated history in ancient cultures across the globe.

Here are the steps for cleansing with sacred smoke:

1   Set an intention to clear and cleanse yourself or your space.

2   Close your eyes and ground your energy within your body, feeling your breath in your chest and abdomen.

3   Connect to the energy of the plant you are working with, and thank it for its assistance and support.

4   Light the leaf or stick and gently waft the smoke around your body or around the room, holding the intention for cleansing and staying fully present.

5   Keep windows closed while cleansing. Once complete, open the windows to release the smoke and the energy it carries.

commercially overharvested. The most sustainable option is to grow and harvest your own plants in a small outdoor or potted garden, but if that is not available to you, seek out organizations that work with local farmers and indigenous peoples helping to ethically grow and harvest these sacred plants.

The following are herbs, plants, resins, and other tools you can use to cleanse your home:

* Rosemary
* Cinnamon stick
* Sage
* Juniper
* Pine
* Palo Santo
* Copal resin

* Frankincense resin
* Dragon's blood resin
* Rosewater
* Chimes
* Crystal singing bowls
* Drums

A great time to cleanse is always around the full moon, the week after your period, after an argument occurred in your home, or when someone is or has been ill in your home, as these are all times we can work with the energy of transmutation and release. Scientific research shows that burning sacred herbs such as sage can transmute and clear up to 94 percent of pathogens in the air for at least 24 hours. So you are cleansing and opening space on many levels!

Where to Place Stones in Your Home

Placing stones throughout your home not only changes the energy of a particular room but can also alter the flow and energy of your entire house, helping to bring more harmony, abundance, and prosperity into your home. Through the principles of geomancy (see "Crystal Grids," p. 51), you can create crystal grids throughout your home to enhance the frequency in your space. Certain crystals can also adjust the overall tones in your house and help to counterbalance the harmful effects of electromagnetic frequencies (EMFs) from technology such as Wi-Fi, wireless phones, and televisions within the home. Below are some guidelines to consider for optimal placement of crystals throughout your home.

BEDROOM: The bedroom should be a calm space for sleep and sex. Certain crystals can be very activating and inhibit deep sleep, so I recommend only bringing one to three stones into the bedroom, focusing on ones that promote tranquility, such as amethyst or lepidolite. You may place stones that are supportive of deep sleep or dream recall on your bedside table or under your pillow. Place grounding stones under your bed or selenite in your windowsills for protection during sleep.

KITCHEN: Crystals in the kitchen can help create a warm and peaceful environment for cooking. Stones such as sunstone, calcite, rose quartz, jade, and carnelian assist in elevating the vibration of a room and bringing in

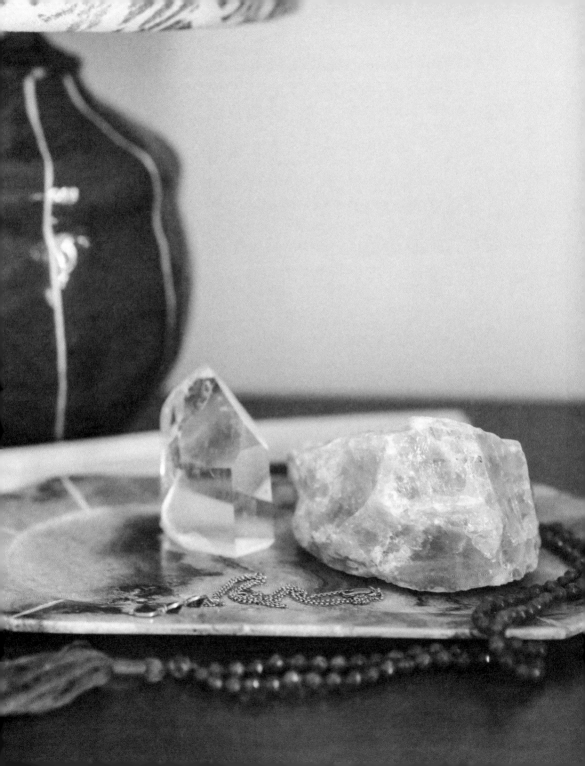

frequencies of love, unity, and feelings of warmth and nourishment. Consider placing grounding and EMF protection stones such as shungite and smoky quartz in areas with electrical outlets or devices.

BATHROOM: Place stones in your bathroom to help facilitate flow—literally and figuratively. Bringing stones into your bath turns your bath into a healing sanctuary. On your counter, place cleansing stones such as kyanite and selenite, or grounding and transmuting stones such as black tourmaline or smoky quartz.

OFFICE: You help alleviate EMF-related issues such as headaches, fatigue, or nausea by placing grounding crystals such as shungite, hematite, pyrite, and black tourmaline near your computer or Wi-Fi routers. Also place howlite, jade, amethyst, and clear quartz on your desk or in your lap as you work to help you stay focused and calm throughout the day.

LIVING ROOM/COMMUNAL ROOM: Stones in your home's communal spaces can help bring feelings of unity and harmony to a group. Place clusters such as clear quartz, amethyst, or apophyllite or larger stones such as rose quartz or citrine in the center of communal areas to help anchor and expand the energy of a room. Also, black tourmaline and petrified wood near the front door can help protect and ground the energy of the house.

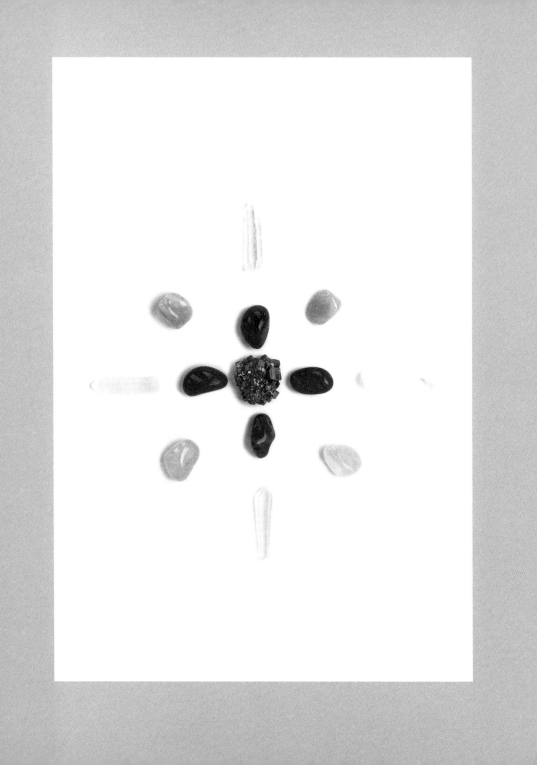

Crystal Grids

Crystal grids combine the energy of minerals and gemstones with sacred geometry, or geomancy, to heighten activation and attunement. They can be used in ritual, manifestation, prayer, as an offering in nature, or as an energy anchor within the home. The following are steps to build your crystal grid:

1   Begin with an intention for your grid and an idea of where you want to place it. A grid in nature might be different from a grid placed in your home. Tune into the energy you wish to create and activate.

2   Select a center stone based on the energy you'd like to activate—this is your main "power" stone—and select 2 to 10 "supporting" stones that energetically align and harmonize with the power stone.

3   Place the supporting stones around the power stone in a structured design. The symmetry and shape of the grid helps to direct and position the energy for amplified power. You may place herbs, flowers, leaves, or twigs around your crystal grid to raise the frequency and collaborate with the energy of the plants as well.

51

Creating an Altar

An altar is a designated area that anchors a particular frequency within a space and helps bridge the material world with the sacred. You might meditate, pray, journal, stretch, or perform your crystal rituals in front of it. It can be a powerful tool to shift and ground energy within you and your home. Ultimately, our true sacred altar resides within—but physical altars activate the sacred in our everyday life and help to consistently bring us back to center.

Each altar is unique, and you can dedicate and decorate it however you wish. Altars can also have an energy of their own. My altars always change depending upon the season, the stones and energies I am working with, and what I am calling into my life. Make sure the energy stays fresh and the altar does not collect dust or have stale flowers. The following are steps you can follow to build your altar:

1   Find an area that can be used exclusively as an altar. It might be a table, shelf, or windowsill.

2   Set an intention for your altar. It could simply be a dedicated space for all your sacred objects or an area where you meditate. You can also be more specific in your intention and create an altar dedicated to a particular goddess or energy, such as an altar for the Divine Feminine or an altar for prosperity.

3   Decorate your altar. You may choose pictures of family members, deities, prayers, candles, feathers, crystals, found sacred objects, or other items of importance.

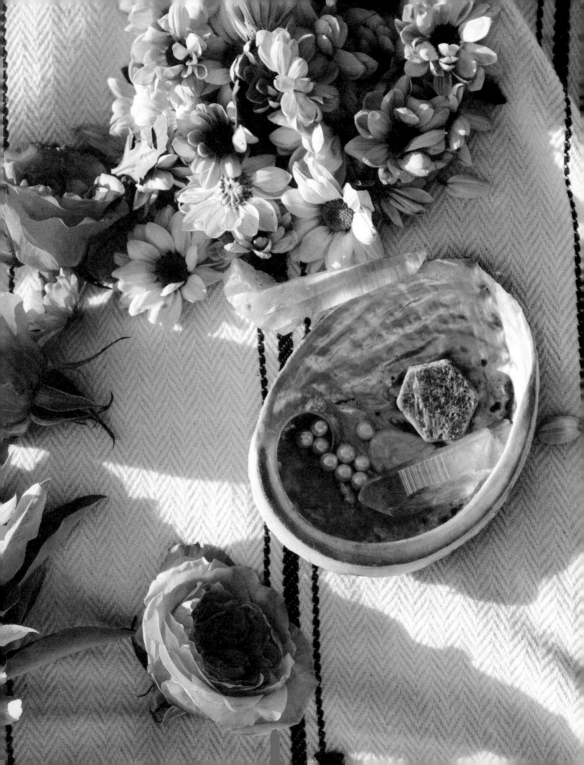

Crystals Wherever You Go

When you engage your crystal for longer periods of time, it anchors that particular crystalline frequency within your electromagnetic field. This in turn helps you to fully acclimate to the healing crystal's tone and ensure lasting changes in your life. When working with particular rituals or manifestation practices, it helps to bring the stones around with you as visual reminders and energetic frequency holders of that which you are calling into your life. Try carrying them in your purse, tucking them into your pockets or bra (just remember to take out before the wash), wearing gemstone jewelry, or placing stones upon your desk at work or in your suitcase while traveling. Crystals are great companions for healing wherever you are.

At Work

Crystals on your desk and in your workplace can heighten your focus, creativity, grounding, and protection. They not only help mitigate effects of EMFs from fluorescent lighting and screens but also help create a harmonizing energetic field with coworkers and bring a sense of calm to your work flow.

CALM: Amethyst, aquamarine, calcite, jade, Larimar, rose quartz

COURAGE/PRESENTATIONS: Amazonite, kyanite, moldavite, peridot, tiger's eye

CREATIVITY: Aragonite, blue apatite, carnelian, ocean jasper, ruby, sunstone

EMF PROTECTION: Black tourmaline, hematite, pyrite, smoky quartz

FOCUS: Howlite, iolite, kyanite, lapis lazuli, pyrite

INSPIRATION/POSITIVITY: Dalmatian stone, Himalayan quartz, kunzite, peach moonstone

Traveling

Even though I have had many bags searched by airport security due to crystals in my carry-on, it is always worth the extra 10-minute wait to have my stones with me while traveling. Crystals can help with anxiety while flying, assist the body in adjusting to new times zones, keep your energy field protected and clear, and help to bring additional luck and flow to your journey. And it also makes me happy to think that the stones are bringing additional healing energy to the airports.

ANXIETY: Amber, chrysocolla, lepidolite, rose quartz, smoky quartz

LUCK: Aventurine, citrine, jade, moldavite, opal

PROTECTION: Black tourmaline, pyrite, selenite, Shungite, smoky quartz

FLOW: Herkimer diamond, kyanite, labradorite, moldavite

Crystals and Chakras

The word *chakra* in ancient Sanskrit translates to "wheel" or "disk," meaning it is a spinning wheel of energy within the body. The chakra system first originated in India, thousands of years ago, first appearing in the ancient yogic literature of the Vedas, linking the physical, psychological, emotional, and spiritual realms.

Although they cannot be seen with the visible eye, you have seven main chakras, or "energy wheels," in your body that receive, assimilate, and express energy as information. Each chakra governs certain principles relating to consciousness and the vitality of life force within the individual. The chakras span from the base of your spine to the crown of your head. When all of these energetic centers are in alignment and healthy balance, there is flow and well-being expressed in all areas of your life. When a chakra's energy becomes out of balance, either deficient or overactive, it signifies that a certain area of your life may require more attention, healing, and care.

The use of crystals in chakra healing and balancing is an ancient healing practice. Crystals hold and radiate a specific harmonic frequency and vibration that helps to bring associated chakras into alignment. When you place crystals on your chakras, your energetic field is able to respond to the vibration accordingly and realigns in harmony and balance.

The Seven Main Chakras

The following is an overview of the seven main chakras and corresponding crystals to heal and harmonize each chakra. Each chakra will express certain attributes when it is balanced and when it is unbalanced.

ROOT CHAKRA (MULADHARA)

AREA OF THE BODY: Base of your spine and perineum

COLOR: Red

CRYSTALS: Black tourmaline, bloodstone, garnet, hematite, Kambaba jasper, petrified wood, Shungite, smoky quartz, snowflake obsidian

WHEN BALANCED: Grounded, safe, financial stability, organized, strong boundaries, healthy immune system

WHEN UNBALANCED: Flighty, anxious, fearful, difficulty with finances, materialistic, greedy, disorganized, cluttered, poor boundaries

SACRAL CHAKRA (SVADHISTHANA)

AREA OF THE BODY: Pelvic region, womb

COLOR: Orange

CRYSTALS: Amber, aragonite, carnelian, moonstone, orange calcite, peach moonstone, ruby, sunstone, unakite

WHEN BALANCED: Creative, passionate, sensual, open to change, expressive, able to express emotions, open to intimate and close relationships, healthy menstruation

WHEN UNBALANCED: Blocked creativity, low sexual drive, unable to express emotions or overly emotional, fear of close relationships and opening up oneself, apathetic

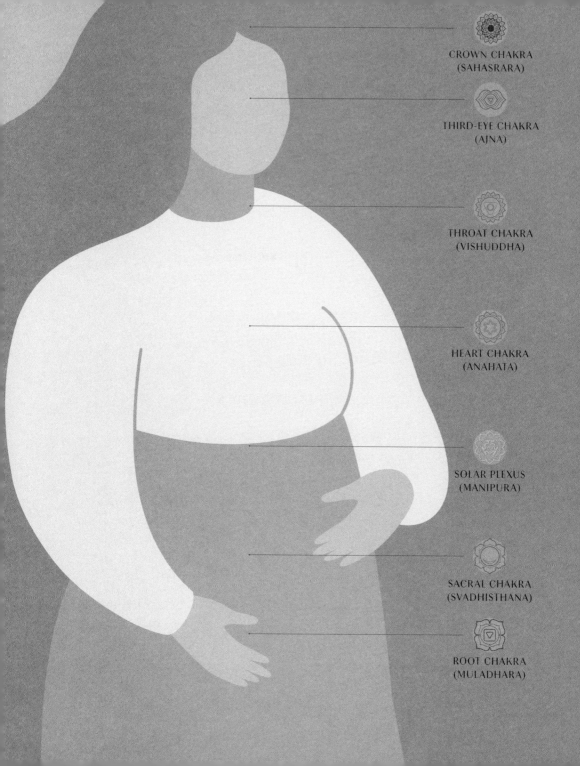

CROWN CHAKRA
(SAHASRARA)

THIRD-EYE CHAKRA
(AJNA)

THROAT CHAKRA
(VISHUDDHA)

HEART CHAKRA
(ANAHATA)

SOLAR PLEXUS
(MANIPURA)

SACRAL CHAKRA
(SVADHISTHANA)

ROOT CHAKRA
(MULADHARA)

SOLAR PLEXUS (MANIPURA)

AREA OF THE BODY: Upper abdomen above navel

COLOR: Yellow

CRYSTALS: Amber, aragonite, citrine, Dalmatian stone, ocean jasper, peridot, pyrite, tiger's eye

WHEN BALANCED: Strong sense of self, confident, strong determination and will, ability to process suggestion or criticism, strong digestion and healthy appetite, follows through on commitments

WHEN UNBALANCED: Low self-worth, victim mentality, feeling powerless, perfectionist, controlling, domineering

HEART CHAKRA (ANAHATA)

AREA OF THE BODY: Center of the chest, heart center

COLORS: Green and pink

CRYSTALS: Aventurine, emerald, jade, kunzite, malachite, moldavite, moss agate, pink tourmaline, rhodochrosite, rose quartz, ruby, ruby fuchsite

WHEN BALANCED: Empathic, compassionate, present, open, feeling loving with nature and animals, peaceful

WHEN UNBALANCED: Intolerant, lack of empathy, codependent, over-giving, negligent to nature

THROAT CHAKRA (VISHUDDHA)

AREA OF THE BODY: Between the collarbone and chin

COLOR: Sky blue

CRYSTALS: Amazonite, angelite, aquamarine, blue apatite, blue kyanite, calcite, celestite, chrysocolla, Larimar, turquoise

WHEN BALANCED: Clear communication of ideas, thoughts, and feelings; creative; great listener; knows when to speak and when to listen

WHEN UNBALANCED: Difficulty getting ideas across, fear of speaking up, not a good listener, gossiper

THIRD-EYE CHAKRA (AJNA)

AREA OF THE BODY: Center of the forehead

COLOR: Indigo

CRYSTALS: Amethyst, azurite, howlite, iolite, labradorite, lapis lazuli, lepidolite, moonstone, opal, pearl

WHEN BALANCED: Intuitive, strong sense of discernment, active imagination, connection with the unseen world, able to process dreams, clear thoughts

WHEN UNBALANCED: Obsessive thinking, lacks trust in one's judgment, overly concerned with physical world, nightmares, inability to use imagination

CROWN CHAKRA (SAHASRARA)

AREA OF THE BODY: Crown of the head

COLOR: Violet

CRYSTALS: Apophyllite, clear quartz, Herkimer diamond, Himalayan quartz, K2, Lemurian seed, moldavite, scolecite, selenite

WHEN BALANCED: Present, wise, strong faith, connection to cosmos, intelligent, neutral, understanding

WHEN UNBALANCED: Judgmental, brain fog, difficulty concentrating, depressed, spiritual hierarchal thinking, dogmatic, inability to integrate life lessons

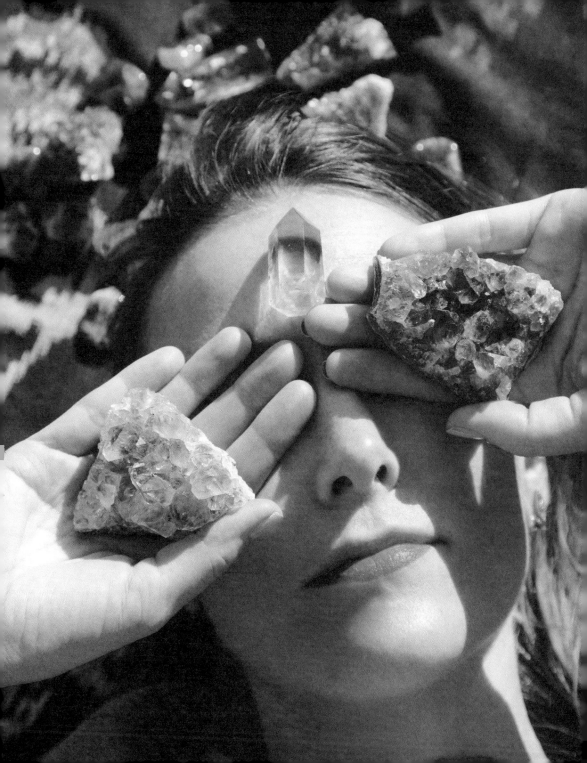

CHAKRA-BOOSTING MEDITATION RITUAL

BEST TIME OF DAY: Morning or afternoon
TIME NEEDED: 15 to 30 minutes
FREQUENCY: As frequently as needed
WHAT YOU'LL NEED: Clear quartz

Our chakras can vary in alignment and radiance depending upon internal and external influences, traumas, triggers, and environmental factors. This meditation brings you back into balance and helps to cleanse, boost, and activate all seven major chakra centers. Use this meditation when you are feeling drained, stressed, unwell, or unbalanced, or use it as a daily or weekly maintenance meditation for overall vitality and alignment.

1 Lie down on your back, and place the clear quartz on the center of your chest.

2 Allow your breath to begin to deepen and lengthen.

3 Set the intention that all seven major chakra centers come into alignment.

4 Bring your awareness to your Root Chakra at the base of your spine and perineum. Envision a bright red spinning wheel moving clockwise. See the red get brighter and brighter. Stay there until the color reaches its peak saturation.

5 Move up to your Sacral Chakra, in your womb. Visualize a bright orange wheel spinning clockwise. Continue deepening the color orange, seeing your Sacral Chakra spin brighter and more vibrant.

6 Bring your attention now to your Solar Plexus beneath your rib cage. Visualize your Solar Plexus as radiant yellow and spinning clockwise. Notice if the color is faint or patchy, and continue spinning the wheel until it reaches a vibrant canary yellow.

7   Now bring your awareness to your Heart Chakra in the center of your chest. Envision a deep emerald green wheel spinning clockwise in the center of your chest. With each rotation, the wheel gets clearer and richer in color.

8   Come up to your Throat Chakra between your collarbones and chin. Visualize a sky-blue wheel of energy moving clockwise, getting clearer each moment. Any dark patches or spots spin off, and the blue becomes brighter with each rotation.

9   Move up to your Third-Eye Chakra in the center of your forehead. Envision a deep indigo wheel spinning clockwise. Each rotation makes the color richer and more saturated.

10 Bring your awareness up to your Crown Chakra at the top of your head. Visualize a bright violet wheel spinning clockwise. Feel it expanding wider and becoming brighter and brighter purple.

11 Stay in this space for a few more minutes. Allow each of your seven chakras to continue to spin in alignment with one another.

12 Take a few deep breaths, and bring your awareness back to the clear quartz in the center of your chest. When you are ready, gently open your eyes.

63

FOUR

Ten Crystals Every Woman Needs

THE CRYSTALS INCLUDED IN THIS CHAPTER ARE KEY FOR every woman. They have been chosen for their individual potency as well as their collective healing power. Together they provide a balanced collection for all seven major chakras and bring vitality, health, wealth, and well-being to life. Most crystals can be paired together to amplify healing and to heighten a specific intentionality. Some of the best pairings feature crystals with different tones that—sometimes surprisingly—greatly complement one another. Similar to building a recipe with different ingredients, a potent pairing can create a healing harmonic frequency that complements rather than clashes.

65

Amethyst

Amethyst is a stone for deep spiritual transformation. It creates an energetic field of high-frequency violet light, keeping your environment protected and clean while also enhancing creativity. Keep it in your meditation or work space to help you stay disciplined and focused on your goals and projects, or allow it to serve as a reminder of your divinity and healing capabilities. I use amethyst pyramids, double terminated points, and tumbled stones for personal healing. Clusters are great to use in communal areas and on your altar at home.

COLOR: Deep purple, purple, pink, lavender

ORIGIN: Africa, Bolivia, Brazil, Canada, Europe, Mexico, United States

ENERGY: Radiates, reflects, amplifies, purifies

CHAKRAS: Crown, Third Eye

PAIRS WITH: Apophyllite, azurite, black tourmaline, citrine, clear quartz, Himalayan quartz, moldavite, pyrite, rose quartz, ruby, scolecite

SPECIAL CARE: Fades in sunlight, so do not place in direct sun for long periods of time.

Manganese and iron give amethyst, a variety of quartz, its distinctive violet color. Amethyst has been revered for millennia as a stone of protection, beauty, royalty, and sobriety (the etymology of its name in Greek means "not drunken"). It was one of the stones on the breastplate of the high priest in the Bible and is connected to the goddess Diana.

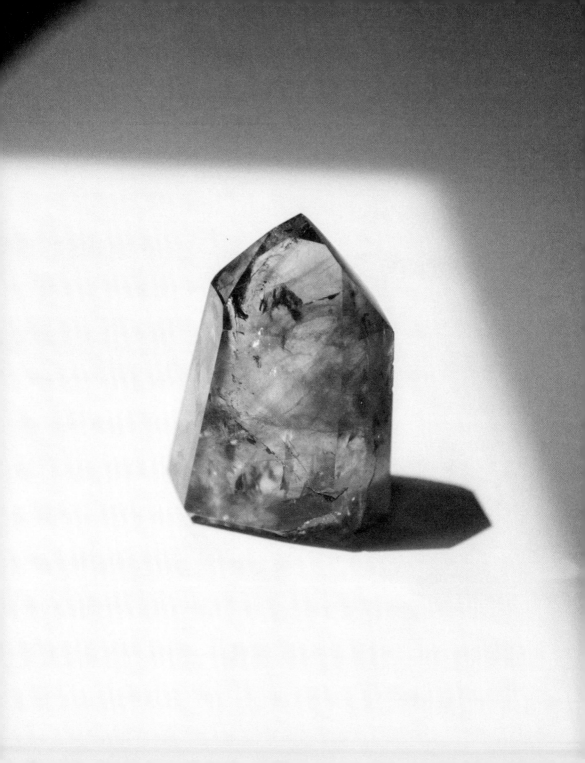

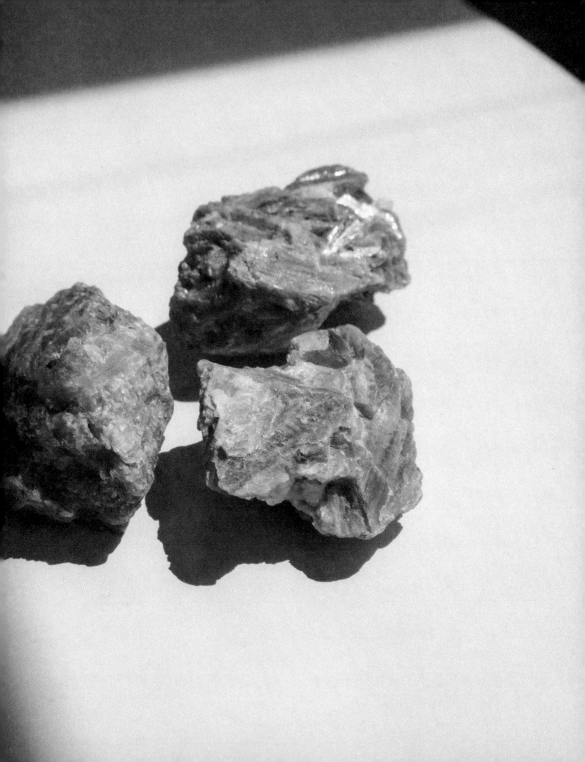

Blue Kyanite

A great equalizer and cleanser, blue kyanite actively transmutes dense energy within a space to keep it clear and elevated. It holds a balance of masculine and feminine energies and allows for these two polarities to flow and harmonize. It helps to heal blockages in the body and imbalances within the Throat Chakra, inspiring you to boldly speak your truth. It is a powerful stone of transformation and rebalancing in its raw form, but it can also be purchased as a comfortable-to-hold tumbled stone.

COLORS: Blue, black, green, pink, white, orange

ORIGIN: Brazil, Burma, Mexico, South Africa, Switzerland, United States

ENERGY: Transforms, balances, cleanses

CHAKRAS: Root, Heart, Throat, Third Eye, Crown

PAIRS WITH: Amethyst, angelite, apophyllite, azurite, selenite

SPECIAL CARE: Kyanite is a self-cleanser and will cleanse and charge other stones around it. It should never be placed in water or salt water.

Kyanite is an aluminum silicate mineral that forms in long, flat edges and is made up of many different layers. While the name comes from the Greek word *kyanos*, meaning "blue," the stone is found in a variety of different colors, including green, pink, and white.

69

Carnelian

Think of carnelian as the spicy chili of the crystal world. It is activating and energizing and activates the sacred sexual energy and prana within. Bold and voracious, this stone enhances creativity, helps you overcome apathy or procrastination, and encourages you to step into your power with courage and gusto. Use it to heal issues relating to the Sacral Chakra, including hormonal imbalances and fertility complications. Look for a tumbled carnelian that you can easily place in your hand, pockets, or in the bath.

COLOR: Orange red

ORIGIN: Afghanistan, Brazil, India, Uruguay

ENERGY: Awakens, activates, energizes

CHAKRAS: Root, Sacral, Solar Plexus

PAIRS WITH: Citrine, clear quartz, garnet, orange calcite, pyrite, ruby, smoky quartz, tangerine quartz

Carnelian is a reddish-orange variety of the silica mineral chalcedony. The name is most likely derived from *cornum*, the Latin name for the semitranslucent cornel cherry. It is believed to have been one of the stones in the breastplate of the high priest in the Bible.

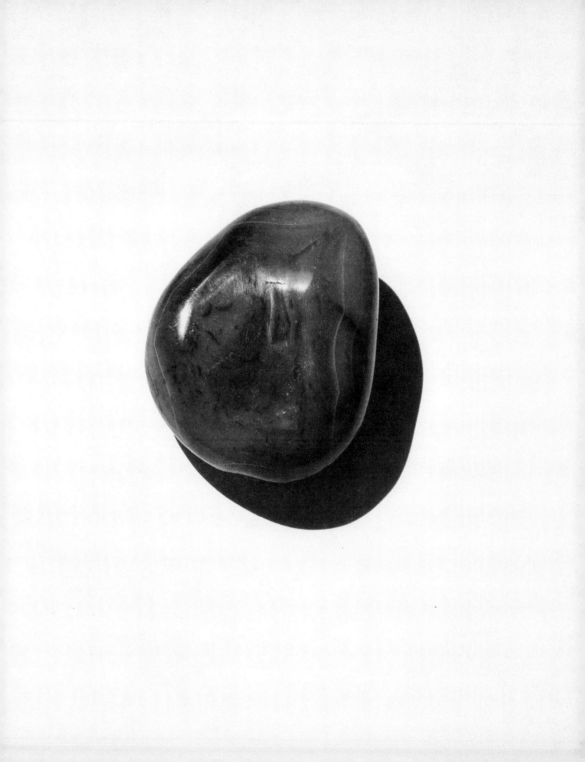

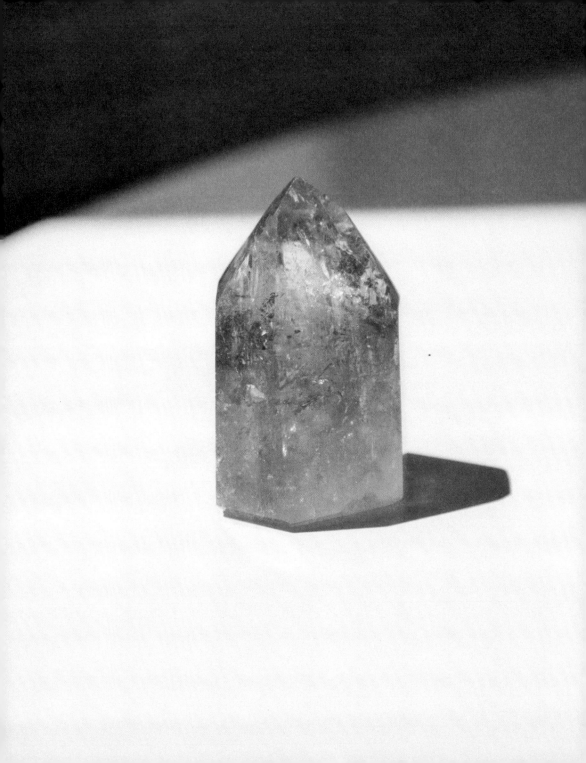

Citrine

Citrine is a stone of personal power. It activates and attunes you to your divinity, abundance, and conscious creator within. Use it to attune to the frequency of prosperity of all kinds, including those related to friendship, health, and wealth. Citrine activates the Solar Plexus and supports the use of power with integrity and consciousness. Natural citrine pyramids are one of my favorite tools for manifestation and crystal grids. Tumbled natural citrine is also incredible for use in healing rituals, meditation, and with mantras.

COLORS: Light yellow to dark yellow/golden brown

ORIGIN: Brazil, France, Madagascar, Russia, Scotland, Spain, United States (California, Nevada)

ENERGY: Amplifies, activates, directs

CHAKRA: Solar Plexus

PAIRS WITH: Amethyst, Herkimer diamond, moldavite, orange calcite, pyrite, smoky quartz

Iron gives citrine quartz its golden yellow coloration. Natural citrine is fairly rare; however, citrine can be created by heat-treating other variations of quartz. Today, most citrine on the market is heated amethyst quartz. Heated citrine may not have the original frequency of a natural citrine, but it still radiates the activating color frequency of yellow and the energies of a golden quartz.

Clear Quartz

Often called the Master Healer Stone, clear quartz could also be called the "master gemstone" as it helps one to energetically attune to all other crystals. It is a highly potent, easily programmable magnifier of energy and intentions and can help you to access and manifest higher states of consciousness. It also amplifies the energies of stones around it. Use clear quartz points in self-healing rituals and crystal grids, and use clusters to amplify the energy of an environment. When placing points on your body, always point the crystal point vertically up and down your body, so as not to break the energy line.

COLOR: Clear, milky translucent

ORIGIN: All over the world

ENERGY: Amplifies, enhances, directs

CHAKRAS: Specifically Crown Chakra, but works with all seven main chakra centers

PAIRS WITH: Most stones

SPECIAL CARE: Needs cleansing often, especially if you notice the clarity becoming murky. Safe to cleanse in water.

Quartz is a silicon dioxide crystal found on every continent in the world and makes up 20 percent of Earth's crust, with 12% on land. Clear quartz is often overlooked because of how prevalent it is, but crystal healers, mystics, and shamans have known for thousands of years that quartz can store, direct, amplify, and hold information.

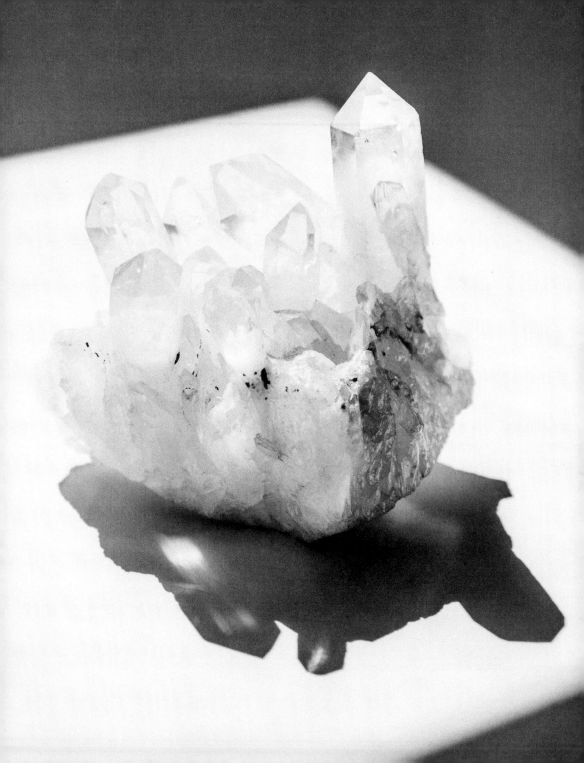

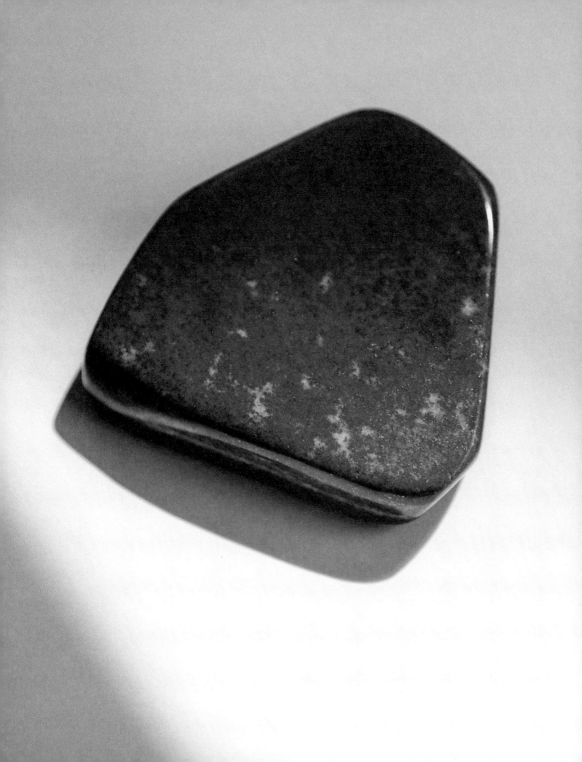

Lapis Lazuli

Lapis lazuli awakens us to deeper insight and connects us with the ancient wisdom of the cosmos. Deeply connected with ancient Egypt, the goddess Isis, Sekhmet, and the ancient civilization of Atlantis, this stone helps us access past lives across cultures and spiritual teachings. It can awaken you to your soul path and purpose in this lifetime, helping to clearly see the helpers, healers, and activators in your life. It is a great stone for meditation, healing work, and connecting with one's ancestors, star beings, and spirit guides.

COLORS: Indigo deep blue with gold veins

ORIGIN: Afghanistan, Africa, Brazil, India

ENERGY: Awakens, activates, directs, channels

CHAKRAS: Crown, Third Eye, Solar Plexus

PAIRS WITH: Azurite, clear quartz, Himalayan quartz, kyanite, moldavite, pyrite

Lapis lazuli artifacts have been found as far back as 3100 BC. Ancient Egyptians used it for jewelry, scarab talismans, and beads. The term *royal blue* comes from this era, when the stone decorated Cleopatra's palace. It has also been ground and made into a paint, as seen in Vermeer's painting *Girl with a Pearl Earring*.

Rose Quartz

Rose quartz radiates the frequency of pure, unconditional love and helps to balance, calm, harmonize, and heal the body, mind, and spirit and deepen the relationship with the self, family, community, and Earth. Tumbled rose quartz is easiest for bath rituals and self-healing meditations. It's beautiful in its raw form as well. I like to sleep with raw rose quartz under my bed and created a crystal grid with rose quartz and flowers for my wedding ceremony.

COLOR: Light pink to deep pink

ORIGIN: Brazil, Madagascar, South Africa, United States

ENERGY: Balances, radiates, harmonizes

CHAKRA: Heart

PAIRS WITH: Angelite, celestite, citrine, Himalayan quartz, jade, Kambaba jasper, Lemurian seeds, malachite, rhodochrosite

SPECIAL CARE: Should not be left in the sun for too long, as it will fade with time.

Rose quartz is a silicon dioxide mineral of the quartz family. Beads of rose quartz have been found from Mesopotamia dating back to 7000 BC. Ancient Egyptian, Roman, and Greek civilizations used rose quartz in talismans and jewelry. It is said medical practitioners in the Middle Ages used it in healing remedies and elixirs. The stone is connected to the goddess Kuan Yin and Mother Mary.

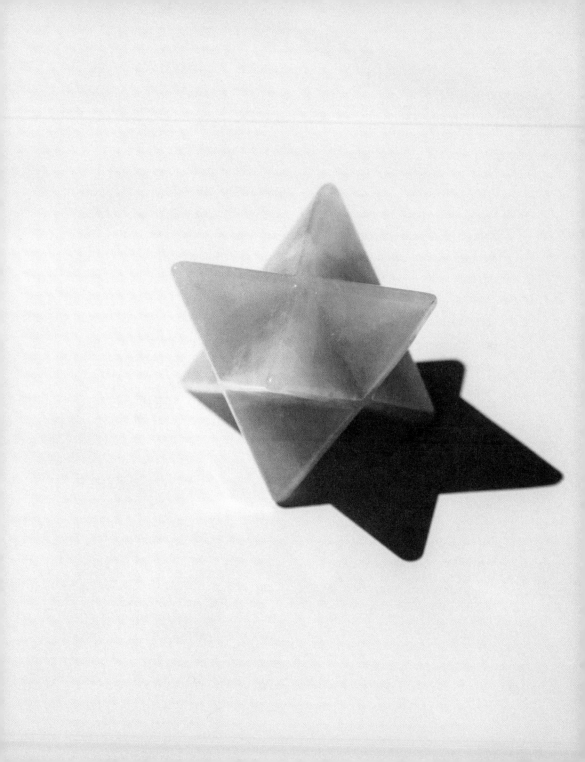

Ruby

Ruby is a stone of passion and the Divine Feminine. Both healing and activating to the Sacral Chakra and Root Chakra, ruby is wonderful to work with for healing traumas of the womb, regulating moon cycles, helping increase fertility, and activating inner strength and the power of sacred sexuality. Ruby is one of the most potent stones for this era of Divine Feminine awakening, and I recommend using small, raw rubies, which are economical and potent, in rituals. Cut and polished forms, including in jewelry, can provide a daily radiance boost.

COLOR: Light red to deep red

ORIGIN: Brazil, Burma, India, Sri Lanka, United States

ENERGY: Activates, awakens, radiates

CHAKRAS: Root, Sacral, Heart

PAIRS WITH: Carnelian, Herkimer diamond, rhodochrosite, rose quartz, ruby fuchsite

Ruby is an aluminum oxide variety of the mineral corundum, and its deep color derives from chromium. In ancient Sanskrit, Ruby was called "king of precious stones." Legend has it that the Chinese emperor Kublai Khan once offered to trade a city for a large ruby. The ruby is often mentioned in the Bible and is connected to Mary Magdalene, Lakshmi, and Aphrodite.

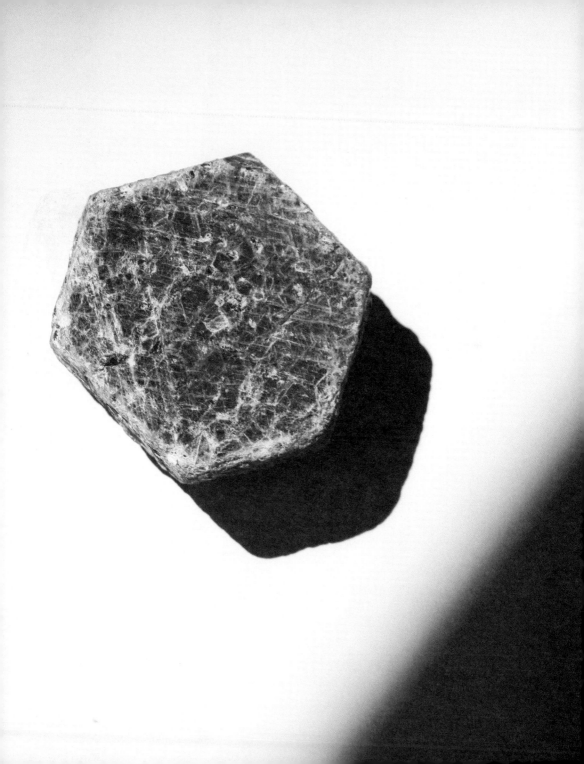

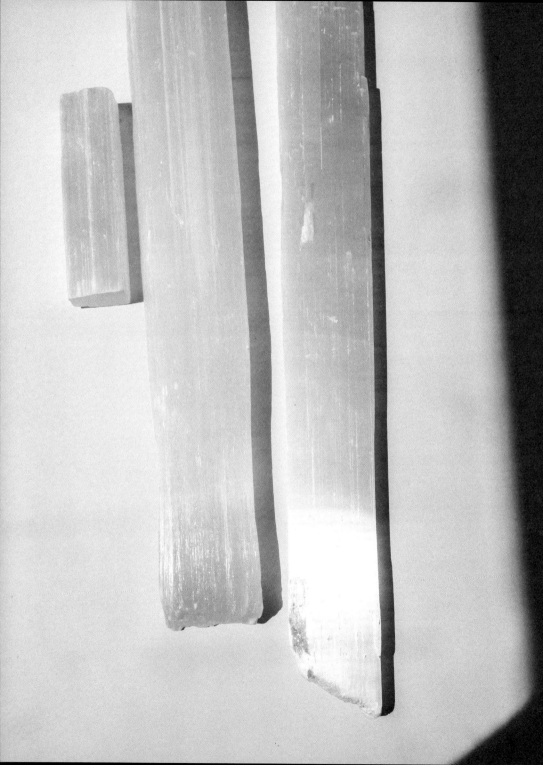

Selenite

A stone of cleansing and activation, selenite quickly and efficiently cleans the auric field while activating the Third-Eye Chakra and opening the Crown Chakra. It's great for healers, teachers, travelers, and medical professionals, as well as empaths and highly sensitive individuals because it can instantly transmute negative energy. Use it at home for self-healing and meditation and to amplify other stones. Selenite wands are generally useful for cleansing and rituals, and I also like to use selenite slabs to cleanse my jewelry and other stones.

COLORS: Clear/colorless, gray, white, green, light brown

ORIGIN: Australia, Greece, Mexico, United States

ENERGY: Absorbs, transmutes, radiates, cleanses

CHAKRAS: Crown, Third Eye

PAIRS WITH: Blue kyanite, moldavite, scolecite

SPECIAL CARE: A self-cleanser, it does not need cleansing. Cannot be placed in or cleansed with water.

Selenite is a form of gypsum, a hydrous calcium sulfate mineral. It forms after water has evaporated near clay beds or around hot springs. Selenite is named after the Greek goddess of the moon, Selene, and is connected to Artemis. While it is a very soft mineral, it is a powerhouse and one of the highest, purest vibratory stones in the mineral world.

83

Smoky Quartz

Smoky quartz helps to transform dense energy while also creating a grounding and calming effect on the system. It is a stone of letting go, surrendering to the unknown, and moving forward in life. Keep it on hand for stressful transitions, such as travel, and use it to maintain high frequencies within a home or communal setting. I love to work with raw smoky quartz points in self-healing rituals, as they direct and move energy quickly. They're also helpful as polished spheres, pyramids, or tumbled stones.

COLORS: Translucent light brown, brown to dark gray/black

ORIGIN: Brazil, Madagascar, Switzerland, United States

ENERGY: Amplifies/absorbs (other terminology)

CHAKRA: Root

PAIRS WITH: Black tourmaline, clear quartz, Shungite, tiger's eye

Smoky quartz is a silicon dioxide mineral of the quartz family. Its color comes from natural radiation emanating from surrounding rocks, which then activates certain impurities within the quartz and gives it a light brown to dark brown color.

FIVE

Crystals
A–Z

THE CRYSTALS IN THIS CHAPTER WERE SELECTED BASED on their integral energetic importance and the healing capabilities that ensure balance and well-being. Some of the explanations and qualities of the following 50 stones are modern interpretations of these ancient minerals; just as humans evolve and our consciousness shifts over time, so too does the way we interpret and work with stones.

Amazonite

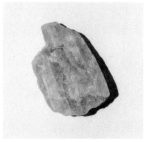

Amazonite is healing and cleansing to the emotional, physical, and astral bodies. It can help you stay grounded within your auric field, creating healthy and supportive energetic boundaries. Amazonite calms the nervous system while stimulating Heart Chakra expansion and activation. It helps you envision the "big picture" of life and see the interconnectedness of all things, rather than getting caught up in the day-to-day minutia. It's a wonderful stone for EMF mitigation as well.

COLORS: Turquoise, blue-green, and green; sometimes with yellow, white, black, or gray portions

ORIGIN: Australia, Brazil, India, Madagascar, Russia, United States (Colorado, Georgia)

ENERGY: Harmonizes, protects, grounds

CHAKRAS: Root, Heart

PAIRS WITH: Aquamarine, aventurine, azurite, black tourmaline, blue apatite, chrysocolla, hematite, smoky quartz, sodalite, turquoise

SPECIAL CARE: Sensitive to heat and chemicals; clean with sacred smoke and charge with selenite or moonlight. Cannot be cleansed with water.

Also called *amazonstone*, amazonite is named after the Amazon River, where large deposits can be found. It's a form of the potassium feldspar mineral microcline. Amazonite is known as a strong stone of protection, wisdom, and nobility. It was found in King Tutankhamun's tomb and used to make 10 BC shields in South America.

Amber

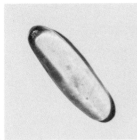

Amber is a warming, grounding, and calming gemstone. It warms the body, bringing vital life force energy to assist with healing of physical pain (including PMS symptoms), injury, or illness. Work with amber to aid fatigue and calm the nervous system. It is often made into teething necklaces to sooth children's pain. It helps bring the element of the warm sun to those suffering from depression, seasonal affective disorder, and anxiety. Amber is a beautiful balance of the feminine energy of Earth and trees and the masculine energy of stored sunlight.

COLORS: Honey, golden yellow, brown to deep brown

ORIGIN: Amber is found all over the world, most famously from the Baltic Sea regions, Mexico, and Tanzania.

ENERGY: Absorbs, transmutes, purifies, radiates

CHAKRAS: Solar Plexus, Sacral

PAIRS WITH: Carnelian, citrine, clear quartz, Herkimer diamond, Kambaba jasper, moldavite

SPECIAL CARE: Do not clean with chemicals or water. Avoid placing in water for long periods of time.

Amber is very soft and easily scratched, with one of the lightest weights of all gemstones. It's a member of the organic gemstone family and is composed of fossilized resin, a substance produced by trees to seal wounds like broken branches. The oldest recorded amber specimen dates back 320 million years. Ancient Egyptians wore amber as an amulet for protection. Stories of amber are found in ancient Greek mythology too.

Angelite

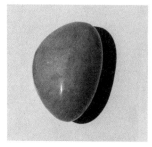

True to its name, angelite is a high-frequency mineral that helps you attune to the angelic realm and your personal guardian angels. It radiates a peaceful, soothing, and calming energy. Work with angelite in meditation, mediumship, and communicating with benevolent souls that have "crossed over," as well as accessing and downloading cosmic universal information. It's an incredible stone for healing on an energetic level, which thus heals on a physical level. Use a tumbled angelite you can place comfortably on the body or in your hands during meditation.

COLORS: Powder blue, light blue, lavender blue, oftentimes with white edges or rusty specks

ORIGIN: Peru

ENERGY: Expands, activates, elevates

CHAKRAS: Throat, Crown, Third Eye

PAIRS WITH: Amethyst, apophyllite, azurite, celestite, clear quartz, jade, sodalite

SPECIAL CARE: A very soft stone, it can be scratched or chipped. If immersed or in contact with water, the molecules will change to that of common gypsum.

Also known as blue anhydrite, angelite is a calcium sulfate mineral. Anhydrite was originally found in 1794, but it wasn't until 1987 that the sky-blue form, "angelite," was found in Peru. Angelite can transform in water, so don't carry it as jewelry or while bathing or sweating.

Apophyllite

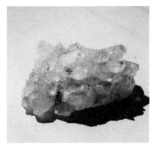

Apophyllite is a high-frequency stone of pure light that can assist you in reaching deep meditative states and strengthening your intuition. This activating stone can connect you to higher dimensional energies such as the star nations, angelic kingdom, Devic realms, and spiritual guides. Its high tone makes it a great crystal for activating the pineal gland, as well as for meditating, setting intentions, and actively raising the dormant life force energy called *kundalini*. Apophyllites are frequently found in a pyramid or cube shape, and they are commonly mistaken for zeolites. Try working with apophyllite in high-trafficked areas of the home or office.

COLORS: Clear, white, gray, green

ORIGIN: Brazil, Canada, Germany, Iceland, India, Italy, Poland

ENERGY: Activates, transmutes, elevates

CHAKRAS: Crown, Third Eye, Heart

PAIRS WITH: Angelite, celestite, K2, kunzite, scolecite, selenite

SPECIAL CARE: Keep out of direct sunlight, and do not immerse in water.

Apophyllite is a hydrated potassium calcium silicate mineral found in clear, white, and gray shades, with the occasional green specimen. Its name is derived from the Greek word *apo*, meaning "off," and *phyllon*, meaning "leaf," because the stone "leafs off" or "breaks apart" when exposed to heat.

Aquamarine

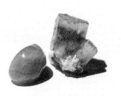

A powerful stone for enhancing one's intuition, aquamarine helps you gain clarity and higher insight and facilitates communication. It is one of the most potent stones to work with for activation of the Throat Chakra and can aid in speaking your truth from a space of integrity and love. Deeply connected to the element of water and the Divine Feminine, aquamarine is an important stone to work with when reclaiming the Divine Feminine energies upon Earth.

COLOR: Ranges from translucent light blue, sky blue, to blue green

ORIGIN: Brazil, China, Kenya, Mozambique, Myanmar, Namibia, Pakistan, Russia, United States

ENERGY: Amplifies, soothes, calms, directs

CHAKRAS: Throat, Crown, Third Eye

PAIRS WITH: Apophyllite, Herkimer diamond, kunzite, Larimar, moldavite, moonstone, morganite, turquoise

SPECIAL CARE: Color fades in direct sunlight after long periods of time.

Aquamarine is a type of beryl, a beryllium aluminum silicate mineral, with a hexagonal crystal system. Found in several shades reflecting the pristine colors of the ocean, its name is derived from the Latin phrase *aqua marina*, meaning "water of the sea." Aquamarine appears in ancient stories as the treasure of mermaids and as a talisman for courage and safety for oceanic sailors and travelers.

Aragonite

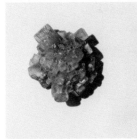

Aragonite aids in releasing outdated modes of being and helps to balance and harmonize the body. It reminds you of the power within and to radiate your true self. Aragonite can help you to stay rooted, grounded, and fully present in your own vibration—which allows you to integrate higher levels of consciousness and energy within your body without getting overwhelmed by outside influences. Work with aragonite to align with your truth, step into personal power, and magnetize your desires into reality.

COLORS: White, red-brown, gray, blue, yellow

ORIGIN: China, Greece, Italy, Mexico, Morocco, Spain, United States (Arizona, New Mexico)

ENERGY: Balances, activates, fortifies, transmutes

CHAKRAS: Root, Sacral, Solar Plexus, Heart, Throat, Third Eye, Crown

PAIRS WITH: Apophyllite, hematite, Kambaba jasper, Lemurian seed, moldavite, rose quartz

SPECIAL CARE: This is a mineral that does a lot of "work" and can benefit from weekly or bimonthly cleansing with water, salt, sacred herbs, or incense.

Aragonite is a calcium carbonate mineral that comes in several colors and forms, the most well known being aragonite star clusters and blue aragonite. Many marine organisms' shells and skeletons, such as abalone and pearl, are actually composed of aragonite or calcite, the mineral forms of calcium carbonate.

Aventurine

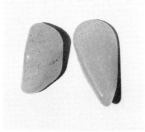

Learn to see the glass half full and find a positive spin to any situation with uplifting, healing aventurine. The stone has been used for good luck and for enhancing one's financial prosperity. Aventurine is a wonderful stone to access the energy of natural abundance, which is reflected in all of nature and the cosmos. It helps to balance both the masculine and feminine energies within, bringing all into alignment and harmony with one another.

COLORS: Green, red-orange, blue, yellow, pink

ORIGIN: Brazil, China, India, Russia, Spain

ENERGY: Amplifies, transmutes, softens

CHAKRA: Heart

PAIRS WITH: Blue kyanite, clear quartz, Herkimer diamond, Lemurian seed, malachite, moldavite, pyrite, rhodochrosite, rose quartz, ruby fuchsite, smoky quartz, turquoise

Aventurine, a silicon dioxide mineral in the quartz family, can be found in several different shades with tiny microscopic inclusions that create a sparkling effect in the light. Allegedly, eighteenth-century glass workers in Italy accidentally dropped copper shavings into a vat of molten glass, creating a glittered effect they called *a ventura*, or "by chance."

Azurite

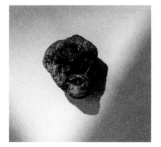

Azurite deeply activates intellect as well as intuition. It helps you to access higher knowledge, insights, and information on a universal level. Work with azurite to meditate, tap into sacred creativity, and increase your intuitive and psychic abilities. The stone can also help access information from past lifetimes and connect with spirit guides. It is often found combined with other minerals; however, when used on their own, the raw small stones are ideal for meditation or carrying in your pocket or bra.

COLOR: Deep blue, often with specks of green from malachite

ORIGIN: Africa, Australia, Mexico, Namibia, United States (Arizona, New Mexico, Utah)

ENERGY: Directs, accelerates

CHAKRAS: Third Eye, Crown, Throat

PAIRS WITH: Chrysocolla, clear quartz, Herkimer diamond, lapis lazuli, malachite, moldavite

SPECIAL CARE: Do not cleanse in water; instead use sacred herbs or resins, or sound.

Named for its deep blue color, azurite was used throughout ancient Egypt and Mesopotamia, and into the Renaissance, as a natural paint pigment. In fact, this is the color that inspired the color "Egyptian blue." Azurite is a copper carbonate mineral that forms in areas where water seeps into copper ores under the surface of the earth, including the large deposit that ancient Egyptians collected near Mount Sinai.

Black Tourmaline

Black tourmaline is a stone of protection and cleansing. It aids in shielding the body and environment from disharmonious and potentially damaging frequencies such as EMFs and heavy, negative, destructive energy or thought patterning. It also helps to ground your body and draw emotional debris down from your body, through your feet, and into the earth. Consider working with black tourmaline to clear energy, including while traveling or working in offices.

COLOR: Black

ORIGIN: Afghanistan, Africa, Brazil, Pakistan, Sri Lanka

ENERGY: Shields, reflects, purifies

CHAKRA: Root

PAIRS WITH: Clear quartz, garnet, hematite, pyrite, Shungite, smoky quartz

SPECIAL CARE: Do not put into salt water or immerse in water for long periods of time. Cleanse with smoke, sound, or selenite, or by burying in the earth.

Tourmaline is a highly conductive mineral that can release negative ions into the air through piezoelectricity (electricity released from friction) and pyroelectricity (electricity released from heating). Also known as schorl, black tourmaline is thought to have been used for centuries by shamans, healers, and alchemists for protection and to clear "negative entities."

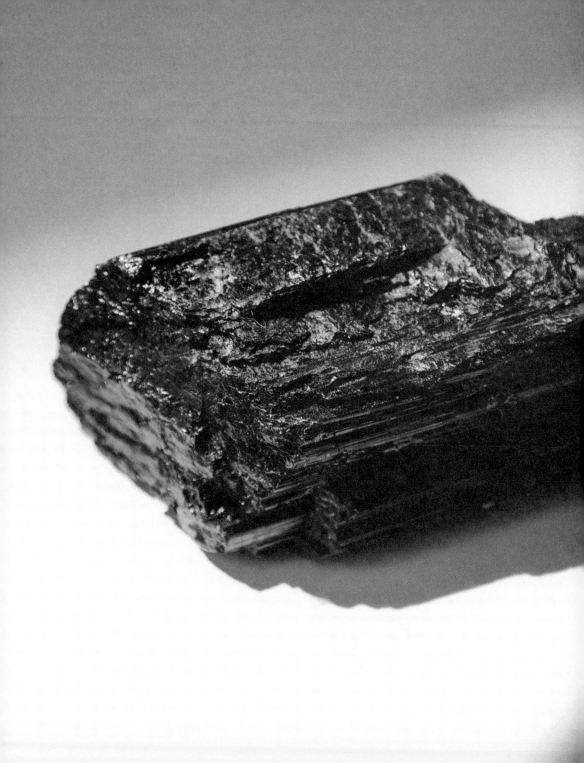

Bloodstone

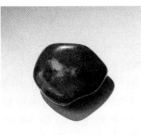

Known as a stone of vitality and movement, bloodstone helps to purify the physical and energetic bodies, releasing heavy, stagnant energy while increasing circulation and blood flow. This stone assists in strengthening your connection to your physical body and sticking to health goals or starting new exercise routines. It also helps you achieve a sense of safety and grounding on the physical plane. Bloodstone can help you find courage in the heart and feelings of internal stability amid change, chaos, or turmoil.

COLOR: Deep green with red inclusions

ORIGIN: Australia, Brazil, China, India, Madagascar, United States (California, Oregon, Washington)

ENERGY: Activates, strengthens, transmutes

CHAKRAS: Root, Heart

PAIRS WITH: Black tourmaline, carnelian, garnet, hematite, ruby, smoky quartz

A variety of chalcedony, bloodstone is formed of green jasper with patchy inclusions of iron oxide. The ancient Greeks believed it bestowed the power of the sun. And, according to lore, bloodstone received its name from the blood of Christ that fell upon the jasper lying at the foot of his cross. It has been historically used as a talisman of protection in battle for increased strength, vigor, and vitality, and as medicine.

Blue Apatite

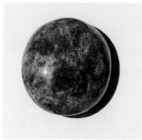

Blue apatite is a stone of intuition and creativity. Its cosmic energy connects you to the energy of the ocean and of the limitless potential within existence, as well as your own infinite creator within. Use it to activate creative energy and to open up the Crown, Third-Eye, and Throat Chakras to connect and communicate with celestial guides and helpers. This stone's vibration connects to the healing frequency of the color blue, the blue cosmic ray energies of Sirius, Pleiades, and the blue light of the Christ consciousness.

COLORS: Blue, yellow, green, brown, gray

ORIGIN: Brazil, Burma, Canada, Madagascar, Mexico, Sweden

ENERGY: Opens, activates, directs, clears

CHAKRAS: Third Eye, Throat

PAIRS WITH: Azurite, blue clear quartz, Herkimer diamond, kyanite, lapis lazuli, moldavite, sodalite

SPECIAL CARE: Do not soak in salt water.

Apatite is the name of a family of calcium phosphate minerals that are commonly found in rocks, bones, and teeth. Apatite receives its name from the Greek word *apatein*, meaning "to deceive or mislead," due to the fact that it can be mistaken for other stones. Many of the moonrocks found from the Apollo programs contain the phosphorous-rich apatite.

Calcite

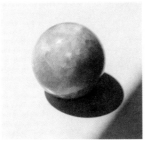

Calcite is both a healing and teaching mineral that can activate the awakening of macrocosmic awareness while harmonizing and restoring your energy field. Each color and variation of calcite can be used for its own specific healing properties. Each of the calcite colors corresponds to a particular chakra: red (Root Chakra), orange (Sacral Chakra), yellow (Solar Plexus), pink and green (Heart Chakra), blue (Throat Chakra), and white (Crown Chakra).

COLORS: Blue, peach, yellow, green, orange, pink, red, white

ORIGIN: Canada, China, Europe, Mexico, Pakistan, Russia

ENERGY: Amplifies, radiates, transforms

CHAKRAS: Sacral, Solar Plexus, Heart, Throat

PAIRS WITH: Apophyllite, blue kyanite, clear quartz, kunzite, rose quartz, selenite

SPECIAL CARE: Can be washed with distilled water, but do not leave the stone in water or cleanse with vinegar.

Best if energetically cleansed with sacred smoke and resin.

Calcite, a calcium carbonate mineral, is found on every continent and even in the human body. Research has found tiny calcite and hydroxyapatite microcrystals on the pineal gland—it is believed that these crystals respond to the electromagnetic frequencies in the environment. Calcium carbonate has also been used for hundreds of years as an acid neutralizer in soil and in medicine.

Celestite

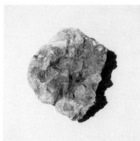

Calming and cleansing to the auric field, celestite is a high-vibrational stone that invokes a feeling of peace, calm, and "lightness." It softens and releases any heavy energy or negative patterning, which allows you to connect to your higher self. Its direct connection with the angelic kingdom assists with increasing clairaudient abilities (the extrasensory abilities to hear beyond the "normal" hearing range) and accessing one's spirit guides and angelic team. Consider placing celestite in children's rooms or gifting them for blessing-ways and other special occasions.

COLORS: Pale blue, white, gray, golden, pink, red brown

ORIGIN: Canada, Germany, India, Italy, Madagascar, Mexico, Poland, United States

ENERGY: Amplifies, absorbs, activates

CHAKRAS: Crown, Third Eye, Throat

PAIRS WITH: Angelite, apophyllite, clear quartz, moldavite, selenite, sodalite

SPECIAL CARE: Cleanse with sound and smoke. Cannot be placed in or cleansed with water.

Celestite, oftentimes called celestine, is a strontium sulfate mineral. It is often mined for its strontium, which is used to manufacture fireworks and refine sugar beets. The world's largest known geode is a celestite that is 35 feet in diameter in a crystal cave in Put-In-Bay, Ohio. According to Greek mythology, celestite is connected to the Pleiades, the star group Seven Sisters, and the companions of Greek goddess Artemis.

Chrysocolla

Chrysocolla is known as the "teaching stone" and "stone of wisdom." It helps ease the mind and calm the body so that you can clearly communicate from the heart. Chrysocolla can also help "detox" or release any physical or energetic impurities your body doesn't need and is a great aid during periods of spiritual growth or transformation. Deeply protective, soothing, and healing to the Heart Chakra, it demonstrates the strength in softness. It's a wonderful stone for creatives, leaders, educators, healers, mothers, and women tapping into their innate wise woman within and leading from the heart.

COLORS: Deep blue, blue-green

ORIGIN: Chile, Mexico, Russia, United States (Arizona, Colorado, Utah)

ENERGY: Transmutes, releases, grounds

CHAKRA: Crown, Third Eye, Heart, Root

PAIRS WITH: Aquamarine, azurite, emerald, lapis lazuli, malachite, ruby fuchsite

Chrysocolla is a hydrated copper silicate and forms in areas of oxidation from the mineral copper. Its name comes from the Greek words for "gold" (*chrysos*) and "glue" (*kollo*) because copper was extracted to solder gold together. It is said Cleopatra carried chrysocolla with her to help ease those around her and to facilitate clear communication.

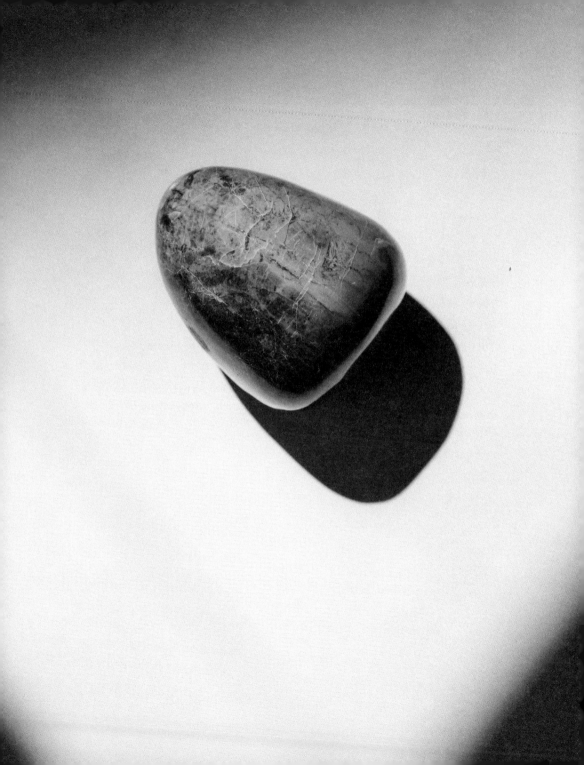

Dalmatian Stone

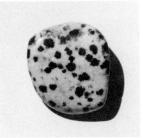

Dalmatian stone is a mineral of play and joy. It reminds you to have more fun in life and not take things too seriously. Incorporate Dalmatian stone into your Inner Child work or to heal childhood or past-life wounds. This stone is also extremely grounding and creates a protective energy within your environment, allowing you to feel safe to communicate and express yourself freely. Turn to Dalmatian stone to boost your self-confidence and bring more enjoyment into your life.

COLOR: Ivory eggshell with black spots and veins

ORIGIN: Mexico

ENERGY: Radiates, grounds, activates

CHAKRAS: Root, Heart, Throat

PAIRS WITH: Black tourmaline, clear quartz, hematite, smoky quartz

Dalmatian stone is often called Dalmatian jasper—but it's not jasper; it's a magnetic peralkaline rock composed mostly of quartz and feldspar. The black spots of the "Dalmatian" are arfvedsonite and are rarely larger than 4 millimeters in diameter. It is named for its resemblance to the spotted Dalmatian dog breed.

Emerald

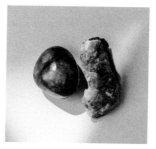

Emerald is a stone of deep love, ancient wisdom, and divinity. It reclaims the self as Divine, aligning you with truth of the heart, alleviating feelings of unworthiness, and bringing you into a state of natural abundance. Honored as a stone of beauty and fertility, this stone opens the Crown Chakra to receive insight and the wisdom to manifest it in the physical world. Work with emerald to step deeper into pure, loving, conscious relationships and to access the ancient lineages of matriarchal leadership. Emerald is connected to the energies of Green Tara, Isis, Venus, Gaia, and Lakshmi.

COLOR: Light green to deep green

ORIGIN: Africa, Brazil, Columbia, Russia

ENERGY: Activates, awakens, amplifies

CHAKRAS: Heart, Crown, Throat

PAIRS WITH: Aventurine, chrysocolla, lapis lazuli, kunzite, moldavite, pink tourmaline, rhodochrosite

Emerald, the green form of beryl, has been revered since antiquity as a stone of power, wisdom, magic, beauty, and high distinction. Legend holds that emerald was one of the four precious stones God gave to King Solomon. In the tradition of Vedic astrology, emerald represents the planet Mercury; in Greek mythology, the Emerald Tablet is said to have been discovered in the arms of Hermes, the messenger of the gods.

Crystals A–Z

Garnet

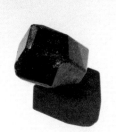

Garnet helps to create your own heaven on earth, grounding your dreams onto the material plane. It connects you to the creative fertile energy of the soil within the deep earth. Garnet activates and heals the Root Chakra and enhances overall vitality. It helps to create feelings of safety and trust within the body, and it can help heal traumas relating to sexuality, safety, abandonment, and rejection. It is a wonderful tool for manifestation and identifying the next steps in any creative process.

COLORS: Red, burgundy, green, orange, yellow, pink

ORIGIN: Brazil, China, India, Kenya, Madagascar, United States

ENERGY: Attracts, anchors, activates

CHAKRAS: Root, Solar Plexus, Heart

PAIRS WITH: Aragonite, bloodstone, carnelian, citrine, moldavite, peridot, ruby, smoky quartz

"Garnet" is actually not a single mineral but is the name given to a grouping of minerals. Although the most common color is red, garnets can be found in a multitude of colors. Its name originates from the Latin word *granatum*, meaning "pomegranate," as a nod to the deep red hue of most garnets.

Hematite

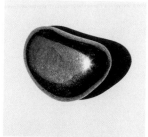

Hematite is one of the best stones for grounding and helps to strengthen a deep relationship with Earth. Work with hematite to find rooting within yourself or if you are experiencing anxiety or confusion from change, transition, or indecision. It is grounding and supportive to the nervous system and blood circulation, making it great for those with anemia, blood deficiencies, or poor circulation. Highly intuitive people often live simultaneously in other worlds or dimensions; hematite helps to anchor the body in the present time and space.

COLORS: Black, steel gray, metallic gray, silver to reddish brown

ORIGIN: Brazil, England, Italy, Morocco, United States (Arizona, Michigan, Utah)

ENERGY: Grounds, strengthens, anchors

CHAKRA: Root

PAIRS WITH: Amethyst, black onyx, black tourmaline, clear quartz, Herkimer diamond, moldavite, ruby, selenite, Shungite

SPECIAL CARE: Do not place in water or salt water, or hematite will oxidize.

Hematite is an iron oxide ore containing 70 percent iron that turns red when it oxidizes. NASA discovered that hematite is one of the most abundant minerals on Mars, which is nicknamed "the Red Planet." Archaeologists have found traces of hematite in ancient peoples from all over the world, starting at 160,000 years ago.

Crystals A–Z

Herkimer Diamond

Herkimer diamonds radiate a very fine, high, pure frequency of light energy and are incredible at amplifying the energy in gridwork, body grids, meditation, and channeling. Herkimer diamonds help to activate extrasensory abilities such as clairvoyance and clairaudience, raise your energetic frequency, and cleanse the auric field. It is a beautiful and potent stone for working with dream time and astral travel, when working with the Akashic Records (the metaphysical vibrational library of all universal knowledge of past/present/future outcomes), for manifesting on the material plane, and for communicating with spirit babies.

COLOR: Clear, colorless

ORIGIN: United States (New York)

ENERGY: Amplifies, radiates, activates

CHAKRAS: Crown, Third Eye, Solar Plexus

PAIRS WITH: Celestite, citrine, kunzite, moldavite, rutilated quartz, scolecite

Herkimer diamonds are silicon dioxide crystals in the quartz family and are only found in Herkimer, New York. They are found in short, double terminated shapes resembling diamonds with glossy, crystal-clear surfaces. Herkimer diamonds are often found with inclusions of black carbon.

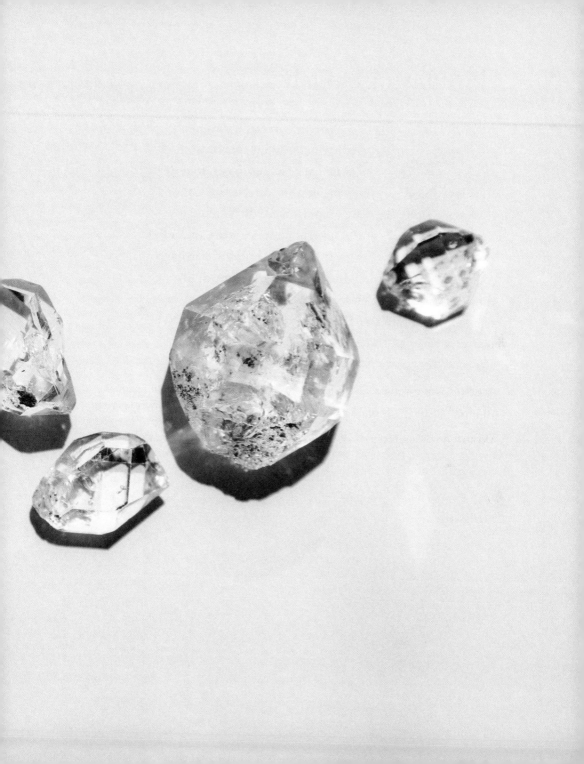

Himalayan Quartz

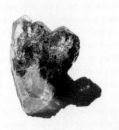

With an extremely clean, high-vibrational resonance, Himalayan quartz is a stone of healing and an ally in times of great change and turmoil. It helps you to access the ancient information stored within its crystalline structure and to see the larger picture of life. Himalayan quartz can clear your energy field, activate and charge other crystals, and boost the overall radiance of an environment.

COLORS: Gray, colorless, blush pink, light green

ORIGIN: Himalayas, India, Nepal

ENERGY: Clarifies, clears, ascends, heals

CHAKRAS: Crown, Third Eye, Heart

PAIRS WITH: Apophyllite, K2, kunzite, kyanite, moldavite, smoky quartz

Called "the Eyes of God" by the Himalayans, Himalayan quartz is an icy, clear type of quartz. These silicon dioxide minerals are found high in the Himalayan Mountains, some 15,000 feet above sea level, and they can be up to 200 million years old. They are said to bring the "yang" or masculine/active energy of the mountain range.

Howlite

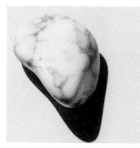

Howlite has a wonderfully calming and soothing frequency. It is a great stone for meditation, especially when just beginning a meditation practice. Howlite has been used to treat pain in the body, strengthen the skeletal system, and balance calcium levels. This healing crystal can facilitate peaceful, calm, clear communication in speaking and writing and is also highly beneficial in treating anxiety and grief.

COLOR: White with gray, black, or brown veins

ORIGIN: Canada, Germany, Mexico, Pakistan, Russia, Turkey, United States (California)

ENERGY: Soothes, balances, releases

CHAKRAS: Crown, Third Eye, Heart, Throat

PAIRS WITH: Aragonite, calcite, celestite, clear quartz, jade, peach moonstones, scolecite.

SPECIAL CARE: Cleanse with sacred smoke and rice, no water.

Howlite is a borate mineral discovered and named in Nova Scotia in 1868. It is highly porous and often found in irregular nodule-shaped forms. Howlite is connected to White Buffalo Calf Woman and is often called "white buffalo turquoise." It is sometimes dyed different colors to imitate stones such as green turquoise.

Iolite

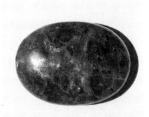

Iolite activates and awakens the Third-Eye Chakra. It helps to assimilate information from one's Highest Self and the Akashic Records (the metaphysical vibrational library of all universal knowledge of past/present/future outcomes) and bring it down into the material plane so that you can put it into action. Work with iolite to organize finances and get out of debt, or turn to it when writing proposals or business plans, and when setting structure to your creative projects. It's also a helpful tool for meditation and aids in awakening dormant extrasensory gifts of clairaudience and clairvoyance.

COLOR: Dark blue to violet

ORIGIN: Brazil, India, Kenya, Madagascar, Norway, Sri Lanka, Tanzania

ENERGY: Activates, awakens, directs

CHAKRAS: Third Eye, Throat

PAIRS WITH: Azurite, calcite (blue), clear quartz, kyanite, lapis lazuli, pyrite

SPECIAL CARE: Do not place or cleanse in water.

Iolite is the trade name of the mineral cordierite, a magnesium aluminum silicate mineral. It gets its name from the Greek word *ios*, meaning "violet," which alludes to its violet-blue coloring. Iolite is known for its pleochroic principles, meaning it appears to change color depending upon the light.

Jade

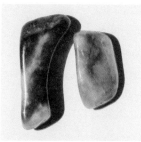

Known as a stone of healing, good fortune, and deep rejuvenation, jade helps you to come into alignment with your highest potential and find the drive to see visions through to reality. It magnetizes helpful people, situations, and thoughts to your energy field when you are ready to step into the next phase in your life. Jade aids in calming inflammation and healing illness within the body. It is a wonderful stone for meditation and active dreaming. It is associated with the goddesses Green Tara and Kuan Yin.

COLORS: Nephrite Jade: white, light green to dark green. Jadeite Jade: purple, black, light green to dark green, lavender, yellow, white

ORIGIN: Nephrite: Canada, China, India, New Zealand, Russia, United States (Alaska, California, Wyoming). Jadeite: Burma, Guatemala, Japan, Russia, United States (California)

ENERGY: Radiates, balances, directs

CHAKRAS: Heart, Solar Plexus

PAIRS WITH: Amethyst, aventurine, emerald, Kambaba jasper, rose quartz

SPECIAL CARE: Best if cleansed with smoke or sounds, not in water.

Jade is a trade name given to describe two distinct minerals: jadeite jade and nephrite jade. Nephrite is a calcium magnesium silicate, and jadeite is a sodium aluminum silicate. Jade has been used since prehistoric periods for carvings, tools, and weapons. It was not until 1863 that a mineralogist discovered that the stone trading across the globe as "jade" was in fact two different minerals.

K2

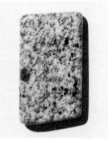

K2 activates and awakens the ancient master within, helping one to access the Akashic Records. It's a beautiful stone for communicating with the angelic and celestial realms, as well as opening up to psychic and clairaudient gifts. Like the energy of a mountain, K2 helps to charge all seven main chakras. K2 is a particularly great fit for those in healing professions and creative professions, as well as soon-to-be mothers.

COLOR: Gray/white, black inclusions with blue patches

ORIGIN: Pakistan (from the mountain K2)

ENERGY: Awakens, activates, strengthens, receives

CHAKRAS: All seven chakras, focusing on the Crown, Third-Eye, Throat, and Root Chakras

PAIRS WITH: Angelite, azurite, Himalayan quartz, kyanite, lapis lazuli, moldavite

SPECIAL CARE: Cleanse with sacred smoke or chimes; do not cleanse with water.

K2 granite is a newly discovered stone comprised of granite made of finely ground quartz, white feldspars, biotite with inclusions of azurite spheres, and malachite specks. K2 is named after the snowy mountain where it is found, on the China–Pakistan border; it is the second largest mountain in the world. Due to the snowy weather and high altitude, mining becomes more difficult, making this stone quite rare.

Kambaba Jasper

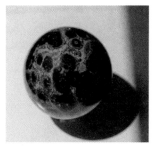

Kambaba jasper radiates the nourishing and rooting energy of nature—specifically wise and ancient tree energy. It can help you slow down, anchor into the earth, and release any unnecessary blockages or stuck energy while drawing up fresh nourishment from your "roots" and into your body. Work with Kambaba jasper to bring yourself back into the pace of nature and feel comfortable in your skin.

COLORS: Blue/gray-green, to deep green with dark stromatolite inclusions

ORIGIN: Madagascar, South Africa

ENERGY: Grounds, calms, strengthens, heals

CHAKRAS: Heart, Root

PAIRS WITH: Black tourmaline, emerald, malachite, pyrite, rhodochrosite, ruby, smoky quartz

Kambaba jasper, also known as *Kambaba stone* or *green stromatolite jasper*, contains stromatolites, or fossilized groupings of blue-green algae, including cyanobacteria that may have helped create the initial oxygen atmosphere on Earth long ago. A stone of ancient beginnings, Kambaba jasper has a strong connection to Mother Earth, the goddess Ostara, and Brigid.

Kunzite

Cleanse your aura and soothe, soften, and expand your heart with a kunzite that radiates unconditional love and compassion. A stone of the Divine Feminine frequency, kunzite connects you to the feminine or matriarchal side of your lineage and to the frequency of the Divine Mother and Our Lady of Guadalupe. It soothes and helps heal old wounds of past relationships and opens you to find the harmony and flow within all of life.

COLORS: Soft pink, deep pink, violet

ORIGIN: Afghanistan, Brazil, Madagascar, Pakistan, United States (California, Maine)

ENERGY: Activates, awakens, radiates

CHAKRA: Heart

PAIRS WITH: Amethyst, apophyllite, Himalayan quartz, moldavite, moonstone, pearl, rhodochrosite, rose quartz, ruby, selenite, tangerine quartz

SPECIAL CARE: Fades in sunlight, best cleansed with selenite or sacred smoke. Do not place in water.

Traces of manganese give this mineral its pink coloration. Story has it that when a large deposit of kunzite was found in San Diego, California, in 1902, the stone was sent to Tiffany & Co.'s gemologist, George Frederick Kunz, who confirmed its identity as a previously unidentified form of spodumene. Kunzite is a high-frequency stone that is part of the collection of "new stones" recently discovered. This stone is supporting the awakening of the Divine Feminine energy on the planet and is important in our evolutionary process.

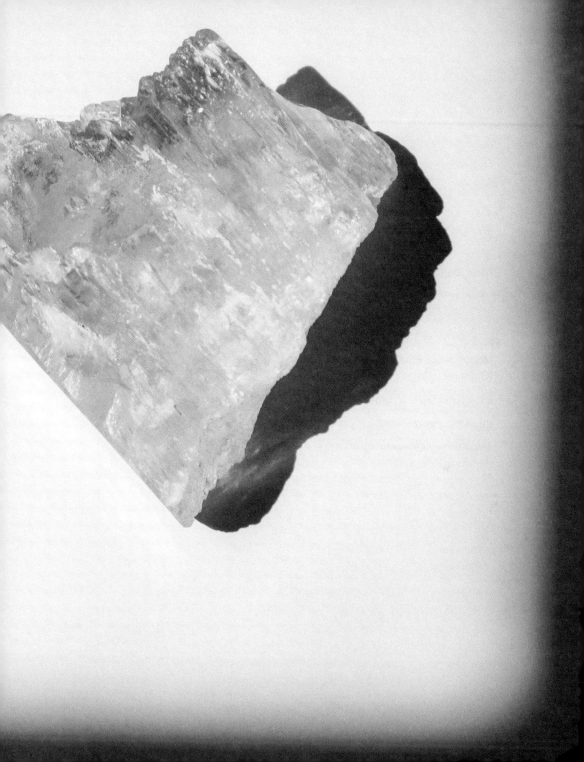

Labradorite

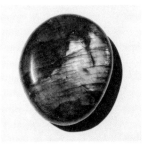

The Merlin of the crystal world, labradorite connects you to the magic within you. It helps you tune into the mystical realm and access the elemental and etheric worlds. Labradorite can help you remember your limitless potential and tap into the frequency of creation. Call upon this stone to create new possibilities, to open up latent gifts of perception and intuition, and to connect with the mystical. Work with this stone during the new moon to bring new possibilities and ideas into form.

COLOR: Green with flashes of gold, blue, purple, and orange

ORIGIN: Canada, Madagascar, Mexico, Norway, Russia

ENERGY: Transforms, connects, protects

CHAKRAS: Heart, Third Eye, Crown

PAIRS WITH: Lapis lazuli, moldavite, moonstone

SPECIAL CARE: Fades in long exposure to direct sunlight.

Labradorite, a sodium calcium aluminum silicate variety of feldspar, was named by Moravian missionaries in the Labrador Peninsula in Canada in the 1800s; however, labradorite was greatly honored by the Eskimo Inuit and the Innu long before that "discovery."

Larimar

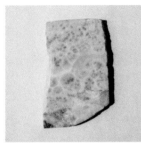

Larimer connects you with the element of water, the ocean, and the wisdom and healing of dolphins and whales. This stone teaches of unity, compassion, unconditional love, and joy. It assists in riding the waves of life, holding space for both the joys and the depths of the soul. This stone holds you within the energy of the Divine Mother and brings you harmony, balance, healing, and deep feelings of safety. Larimar is associated with Yemaya, the African goddess of the ocean.

COLOR: Robin-egg blue

ORIGIN: Dominican Republic

ENERGY: Transmutes, activates, awakens

CHAKRAS: Throat, Heart

PAIRS WITH: Apophyllite, azurite, blue apatite, kyanite, lapis lazuli

SPECIAL CARE: Can be placed in water; great stone to cleanse in the ocean or a body of water.

Larimar is a blue variety of pectolite, a sodium calcium silicate found only in and around the Dominican Republic in the Caribbean Ocean. Often called "the Stone of Atlantis," Larimar was made well known by the clairvoyant Edgar Cayce, who predicted a blue stone of great healing potential would be found in the area.

Crystals A–Z

Lemurian Seed

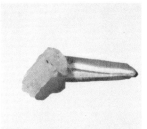

Lemurian seed crystals hold the vibration and frequency of the ancient civilization of Lemuria, reminding us at this time in our history to return to the heart, the frequency of harmony, and the oneness with nature and one another. Lemurian seeds hold a high, fine frequency that's ideal for healing, meditation, and awakening to your unique gifts. They remind you of your soul path, your mission and purpose to reawaken to your own divinity. These crystals also hold the frequency of dolphins, reminding you of your unique imprints and gifts within the whole collective.

COLOR: Clear, soft pink hue

ORIGIN: Brazil, Columbia

ENERGY: Awakens, activates, integrates

CHAKRAS: Root, Heart, Crown

PAIRS WITH: Kunzite, Larimar, peach moonstone

A unique form of clear quartz, Lemurian seed was discovered in Brazil in 1999. These stones have ridges along their sides that are often called the "stairwell to heaven." It is thought that by meditating and rubbing the grooves on these crystals, you can access the information coded by the Lemurian civilization, much like reading a book.

Lepidolite

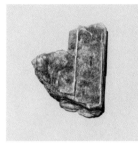

Find deep peace and a calming of the mind with lepidolite. Often referred to as the "Xanax of the mineral world," this stone soothes and relaxes frayed emotions, an overworked mind, and a tense physical body. It can calm the central nervous system and is a wonderful stone for when you feel anxious or overwhelmed, or if coping with panic disorder, insomnia, and PMS. Lepidolite can support deep restoration and balance of body and spirit.

COLOR: Lavender-gray, pink, yellow, gray

ORIGIN: Africa, Brazil, Greenland, United States

ENERGY: Absorbs, soothes, calms

CHAKRAS: Heart, Third Eye

PAIRS WITH: Amethyst, kunzite, pink tourmaline, rose quartz, scolecite, smoky quartz

SPECIAL CARE: Do not place in water or salt water.

Lepidolite is a member of the mica family, a potassium lithium aluminum silicate. It is the most lithium-abundant mineral, causing it to be deeply relaxing and calming. It is named after the Greek word *lepidos*, meaning "flake," because of the stone's tendency to flake off. Trace amounts of manganese give it a range of hues.

Malachite

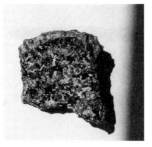

Malachite offers protection, deep healing, and cleansing on both physical and energetic levels. This stone helps to release old traumas, wounds, and patterns stored within the cellular structure of the body and is a beautiful stone to work with in times of transition, heartbreak, and loss. Malachite helps release harmful energetic patterning from one's field while strengthening and activating the electromagnetic field of the heart. This powerful restructure helps you move through challenging periods with grace and determination.

COLOR: Light green to dark green

ORIGIN: Australia, Germany, Italy, Mexico, Namibia, Russia, South Africa, United States

ENERGY: Transmutes, protects, cleanses, activates

CHAKRAS: Heart, Root

PAIRS WITH: Azurite, chrysocolla, kyanite, smoky quartz, tiger's eye, turquoise

SPECIAL CARE: Tumbled malachite can go in water; raw stones cannot.

Ancient Egyptians treasured malachite, a copper carbonate mineral, and used it in jewelry, makeup, paint, and art. Cleopatra was known for creating a malachite-lined eyeliner. Protective malachite has also been found in the castle walls of Russian czars, throughout Italy, and in ancient Aztec artifacts.

Moldavite

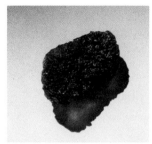

Moldavite is one of the most powerful tools of transformation. Not for the faint of heart, this stone will help facilitate a complete restructure if called to. It accesses the soul's DNA, ancestral karmas, Akashic Records, and the universal codes of consciousness and is associated with communication with entities not of this planet. It is a highly charged stone, helping to dramatically boost the energies of other stones and the environment. Slowly introduce this stone into your life so that you can adjust your frequency accordingly.

COLOR: Pale green to dark green

ORIGIN: Czechoslovakia

ENERGY: Accelerates, amplifies, transforms

CHAKRAS: Heart, Root, Crown

PAIRS WITH: Apophyllite, aquamarine, lapis lazuli, rose quartz, scolecite

SPECIAL CARE: Self-cleanser and self-charger, but can use sacred smoke or tones if needed.

One of the only stones not of this earth, moldavite is a green tektite created by a meteorite hitting Earth 14.7 million years ago in what is now southern Germany. Some people believe the heat created the stones while others believe they are extraterrestrial in origin.

Crystals A–Z

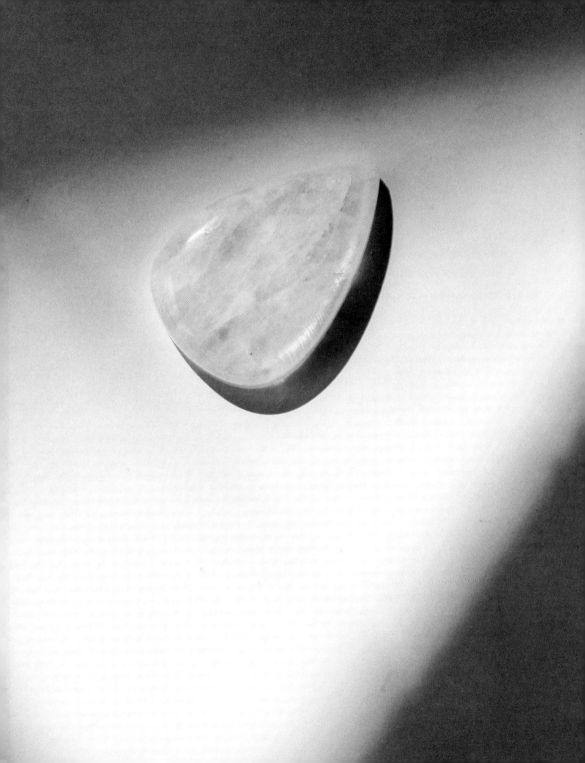

Moonstone

Moonstone is the stone of new beginnings and connects you to the Divine Feminine energies of the moon, the lunar cycles within your body, and all of life. Moonstone radiates the frequencies of the Maiden, Mother, and Crone, yet reminds us that even as we go through these different phases in our lives, we are all of them simultaneously. Moonstone can help connect you to deeper levels of intuition and insight and show you to trust your own intuitive powers over anything else.

COLORS: Colorless with blue sheen, peach, gray, pink, yellow, brown, green

ORIGIN: Australia, Burma, India, Madagascar, Sri Lanka, United States

ENERGY: Projects, amplifies, balances

CHAKRAS: Crown, Third Eye

PAIRS WITH: Apophyllite, labradorite, peach moonstone, selenite

Moonstone, a mineral of the feldspar group, has been long revered as a stone of the goddess energies and related to the energies of the moon. Because of its unique structure, as light passes through the stone, it appears to change color. Moonstone is associated with Freya, Isis, Artemis, Brigid, and Ixchel.

Moss Agate

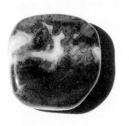

Earthy, nourishing, and grounding, moss agate is a stone of pleasure and harmony on the physical plane. It helps you to tune into the energies of nature and Mother Earth and assists with healing wounds of the heart and traumas relating to your childhood and mother. It helps you access the healing frequency of forgiveness. As it attunes to deep feminine wisdom held within the body, it is a wonderful stone to help increase fertility and support you in staying grounded and present during childbirth.

COLOR: Clear with green, blue, or brown inclusions

ORIGIN: Brazil, France, India, Italy, United States, Uruguay

ENERGY: Connects, anchors, calms

CHAKRAS: Root, Heart

PAIRS WITH: Angelite, clear quartz, jade, Kambaba jasper, malachite, smoky quartz

Moss agate is technically a chalcedony with dendrite inclusions, not a true banded agate. The inclusions resemble moss or lichen growing over vegetation, which is where it gets its name. European farmers were known to hang moss agate beads and pieces over fences, in trees, and even over their oxen to increase fertility of planting for successful harvests.

Ocean Jasper

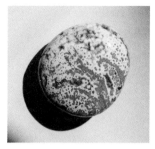

Each unique and colorful piece of ocean jasper reminds you that you need not limit or keep yourself small in order to thrive. Instead you can be bold and brave and create in alignment with your heart and true self.

Ocean jasper radiates the vast creative potential within us all. It stimulates joy and self-expression and releases stagnancy or fears of being seen. It's a wonderful stone for children and adults who wish to access the playful child within them.

COLORS: White, green, orange, blue, yellow, brown

ORIGIN: Madagascar

ENERGY: Activates, awakens, opens

CHAKRAS: Solar Plexus, Heart, Sacral, Throat

PAIRS WITH: Calcite, malachite, moldavite

Ocean jasper only comes from one place in the world: Madagascar. It is a member of the quartz group and can be found in a wide array of colors and patterns. In 2009, the original source was depleted and mining stopped. The stone is rare, but you can still find it available for purchase.

Opal

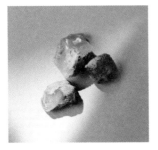

Connect to the frequency of rainbow light with opal to align and heal all seven major chakras and energy centers. Opal bathes the wearer in protective light, making it particularly good for highly sensitive individuals and children. It can expand creativity, calm the mind, and help you access your own unique gifts and potentials within. Opal can bring you to higher levels of intuition and insight while providing energy to manifest on the physical plane.

COLORS: White, blue, black, pink, fire

ORIGIN: Australia, Ethiopia, Mexico, United States

ENERGY: Radiates, activates, attunes

CHAKRAS: All seven chakras

PAIRS WITH: Amethyst, blue kyanite, emerald, kunzite, moonstone, pearl, selenite

Opal is hydrated silica that can contain as much as 20 percent water within its structure. Rich in history and lore, opal get its name from the Sanskrit word *upala* and the Latin word *opalus*, both meaning "precious stone." The Romans believed opal to be the most powerful stone of all. It has long been seen as a stone of luck, hope, and protection.

Peach Moonstone

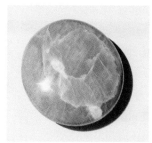

Soothing, calming peach moonstone is wonderful for pregnancy and childbirth, as well as for highly sensitive and intuitive children. Its loving presence calms worries and an overactive mind. Work with it in meditation and restorative baths or to help you see the positive side in aspects of life. Carry a tumbled peach moonstone or "worry stone" in your pocket or purse throughout the day to help ease anxiety and create a balanced, peaceful energetic field.

COLOR: Light peach to golden orange

ORIGIN: Brazil, India, Sri Lanka, United States

ENERGY: Attunes, reflects, strengthens

CHAKRAS: Sacral, Heart

PAIRS WITH: Lemurian seeds, lepidolite, moonstone, rose quartz

Peach moonstone is a unique colorway of moonstone with inclusions of iron. The mineral grouping feldspar makes up 50 percent of Earth's crust. A stone of the high priestess, peach moonstone attunes to the Divine Feminine energies present in moonstone and affirms your true self.

Pearl

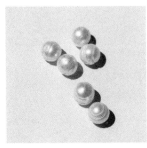

One of the best-loved gemstones of all time, pearl connects to your own gems within. It can help you see the wisdom held deep inside you, especially lessons learned in difficult situations; it will call upon you to act in swiftness, integrity, grace, and softness, even in the face of challenge or uncertainty. It's especially suitable for pregnancy and childbirth, as it possesses a deeply feminine and mothering energy and serves as a reminder of the gift of the "jewel" that is received upon birth.

COLORS: White, yellow, gray, blush, pink, lavender, black, blue

ORIGIN: Australia, China, French Polynesia, Japan

ENERGY: Integrates, softens, enhances

CHAKRAS: Third Eye, Crown, Sacral

PAIRS WITH: Clear quartz, opal, scolecite

Pearls are made of the same substances found in minerals such as aragonite and calcite, but they are created inside the soft tissue of living mollusks. Each natural pearl is unique in shape and size. Wild pearls were once so rare and expensive that Pierre Cartier traded a double strand of pearls in 1917 for a Fifth Avenue mansion in Manhattan.

Peridot

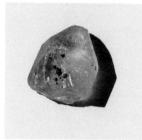

Peridot radiates the energy of unconditional love and divine abundance. The Earth, Gaia, is naturally abundant; peridot reminds us of the inherent abundance and beauty within us all. Peridot can assist in radiating gratitude, staying open and present, and seeing the hidden potentialities for growth and expansion along your path. It helps you see each situation as an opportunity and every person as a guide, teacher, and healer.

COLOR: Olive green to lime green

ORIGIN: Australia, Brazil, Pakistan, South Africa, United States

ENERGY: Radiates, activates, strengthens

CHAKRAS: Solar Plexus, Heart

PAIRS WITH: Citrine, emerald, moldavite, pyrite, tiger's eye

Also called olivine, peridot is a magnesium iron silicate mineral with a lime-green color. Some Egyptian peridot artifacts date back to 2,500 years ago, and some Greek and Roman peridot beads date back to the third century. Peridot possesses the energy of the sun and connects to the goddess Lakshmi and Mother Earth.

Petrified Wood

A stone of patience and support, petrified wood carries the energy of the ancient and wise trees from which it originated millions of years ago. This fossilized wood (often called *agatized wood*) reminds you to come back into harmony with nature and gently anchors energy into the earth while still allowing for expansion and cosmic connection. Empaths, highly sensitive individuals and children in particular may find it to be grounding and supportive.

COLORS: Brown, black, gray, yellow, red, violet, orange, blue

ORIGIN: Argentina, Australia, Canada, China, Ecuador, Egypt, United States

ENERGY: Anchors, activates, awakens

CHAKRAS: Root, Heart, Third Eye, Crown

PAIRS WITH: Bloodstone, clear quartz, Herkimer diamond, Kambaba jasper, Lemurian seed, moldavite, pyrite

Petrified wood is a form of quartz that has formed over millions of years. The process of fossilization occurs when a tree dies and is buried in sedimentary material. Over time, mineral-laden water replaces the wood and crystallizes, preserving the shape, structure, and rings of the tree long after it's gone.

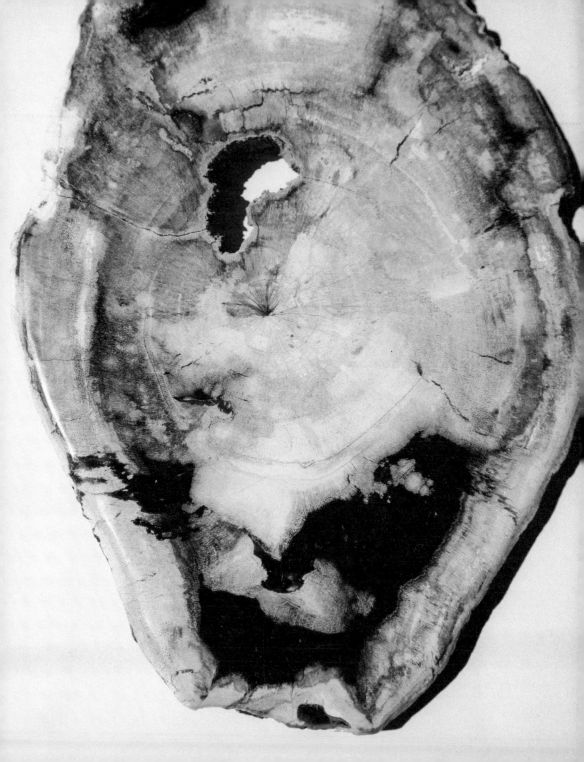

Pink Tourmaline

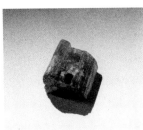 With a beautiful, warming, and calming presence, pink tourmaline cleanses the Heart Chakra, releasing stagnant energy while gently activating and opening the heart. It is the stone of the Divine Feminine, is associated with the planet Venus and Pink Ray of Light, and relates to the Maiden, Mother, Enchantress, and Crone archetypes. It can be a fantastic addition to your self-care and love rituals for women of all ages and stages of life. With its high healing frequency to the heart, pink tourmaline is a beautiful stone to channel unity, unconditional love, and forgiveness.

COLOR: Light pink to deep magenta

ORIGIN: Africa, Brazil, United States

ENERGY: Absorbs, transmutes, radiates

CHAKRAS: Heart, Sacral

PAIRS WITH: Kunzite, lepidolite, rhodochrosite, rose quartz, ruby, ruby fuchsite

SPECIAL CARE: Do not place in salt water, can be cleansed in water but not immersed for long periods of time.

Tourmaline is found in many different varieties and colors, but pink tourmaline is only available in shades of pink ranging from pale pink to almost red. It is thought that the Russian crown jewels are in fact deeply toned pink tourmaline, not rubies. Tourmaline is also associated with Mary Magdalene, Mother Mary, and Isis.

Pyrite

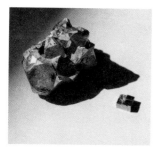

Pyrite brings a masculine energy of structure and the sun. It helps act as a shield and protector from unwanted negative energies and harmful EMFs, and it also helps to create structure and drive in your life. Work with pyrite to channel the focus and determination you need to manifest abundance and realize your dreams. It is an incredible stone for magnetizing intentions and boosting the energy within a home and office. It's available in clusters and natural cubes, which are ideal for crystal grid placement and self-healing.

COLOR: Metallic gold

ORIGIN: Italy, Peru, Spain

ENERGY: Directs, protects, amplifies

CHAKRAS: Solar Plexus, Root

PAIRS WITH: Azurite, black tourmaline, clear quartz, Herkimer diamond, lapis lazuli, Lemurian seed, malachite, Shungite

SPECIAL CARE: Do not place in water. Cleanse with smoke, sound, or selenite.

Pyrite is an iron sulfide mineral that comes in cubic, octahedral, and pyritohedral forms. Its name comes from the Greek word for "fire" (*pyr*) because you can create a spark by striking two pieces of it together. In addition to creating fire, it was used in early firearm devices. Often referred to as "fool's gold," pyrite was mistaken for gold during the Gold Rush.

135

Rhodochrosite

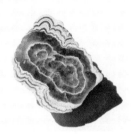

Rhodochrosite is an incredibly powerful heart-healing stone. It creates a gentle opening for stored traumas and wounds within the heart to surface, integrate, and heal, while emanating a warmth and loving vibration. It reminds you that change is the constant in life and to stay open and present while in the midst of transition. This is a great stone to work with while moving through relationship breakups or conscious uncoupling, as it can bring the focus of your energy back to self-love and of healing the heart.

COLOR: Pink, ranging from light pink to magenta

ORIGIN: Argentina, United States

ENERGY: Amplifies, radiates, strengthens

CHAKRA: Heart

PAIRS WITH: Aventurine, clear quartz, emerald, Kambaba jasper, rose quartz, ruby, ruby fuchsite

Rhodochrosite is a manganese carbonate mineral. The gradation of pink tones depends upon the amount of iron, calcium, and magnesium present. Large deposits were found in an abandoned Incan silver mine in Argentina in the 1300s, giving it the nickname "Inca Rose." Rhodochrosite is connected with Mother Mary.

Ruby Fuchsite

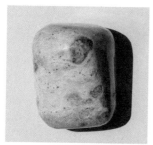

Ruby fuchsite is a stone of healing and cleansing. It brings one into energetic balance and strengthens and activates the emotional body. It helps release old wounds, allowing you to process them and let them go. **This release helps open the way for the vitality of ruby fuchsite to come in and create from a space of grounded presence. It's a wonderful stone for the heart and helps you find the courage to go after your dreams.**

COLORS: Green, white; both with red inclusions

ORIGIN: India

ENERGY: Amplifies, releases, activates

CHAKRAS: Root, Heart

PAIRS WITH: Aventurine, garnet, ruby, tourmaline

Ruby fuchsite is a naturally occurring combination of ruby and green fuchsite that's found only in South India. Fuchsite is a mica mineral and is extremely protective. With the ruby inclusions, ruby fuchsite is a powerful stone to increase your strength and vigor while cleansing the emotional body.

Scolecite

Scolecite is a very high-vibrational stone of pure light. This stone helps you to access any extrasensory gifts that may be dormant, awakening and strengthening the gifts of clairaudience, clairvoyance, clairsentient, and claircognizance. Since it opens the Third-Eye and Crown Chakras, scolecite is a great stone to strengthen your meditation practice daily. It helps to activate the pineal gland, and you might feel a gentle tapping on the middle of the forehead when holding this stone.

COLORS: White, colorless, pale pink, green, peach

ORIGIN: Iceland, India

ENERGY: Activates, awakens, ascends

CHAKRAS: Crown, Third Eye

PAIRS WITH: Apophyllite, clear quartz, selenite

SPECIAL CARE: Do not place in water.

Scolecite is a hydrated calcium aluminum silicate that occurs in both vertical prismatic crystals and fibrous crystal masses. It is generally colorless or white and can have a milky yellow hue. It is known as the "kundalini stone," as it helps awaken the kundalini life force energy within.

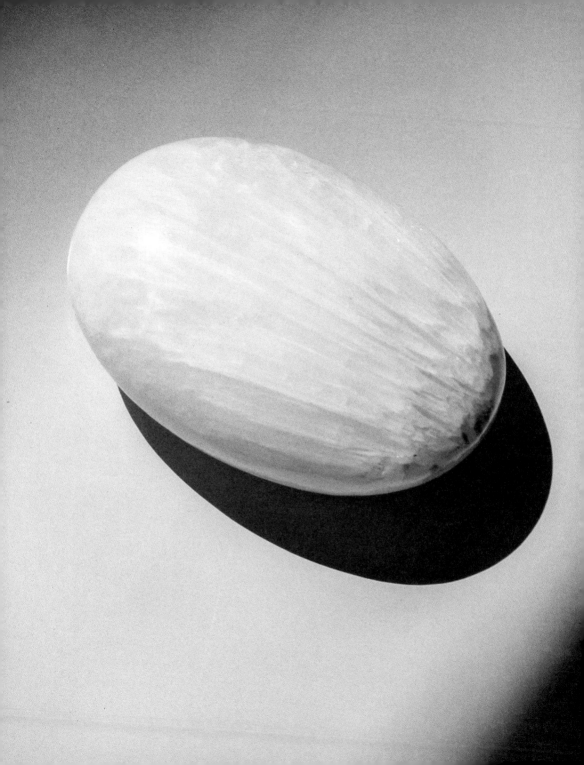

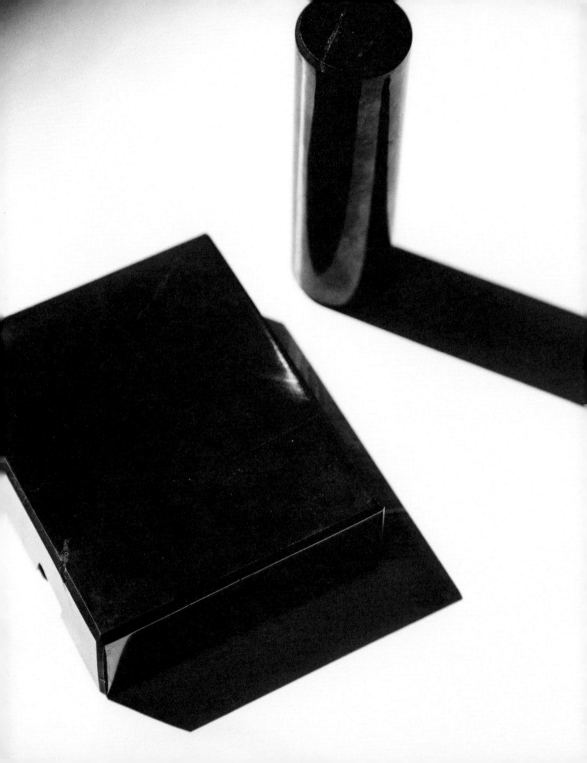

Shungite

Shungite is an incredible stone for energetic release, as well as for cleansing and detoxifying your physical space. It is one of the best stones for mitigating the effects of EMFs. Place Shungite by Wi-Fi routers, computers, television screens, and security systems to absorb and transform the energy of the space. Also consider working with Shungite while traveling or after spending long periods of time at the computer.

COLOR: Dull dark gray to dull black

ORIGIN: Russia

ENERGY: Absorbs, cleanses, transmutes

CHAKRA: Root

PAIRS WITH: Black tourmaline, pyrite, smoky quartz

SPECIAL CARE: Shungite is one of the rare stones that does not require cleansing, but instead can help cleanse other stones. It is safe to use with water.

Shungite is a noncrystalline mineraloid consisting of 98 percent carbon, giving it electroconductive properties and certain chemical resistance. It has long been used to cleanse water and disinfectant. It is said that Peter the Great made sure each soldier carried a stone with them to clean wounds and purify water.

Snowflake Obsidian

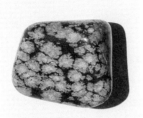

**Often called a "stone of purity,"
snowflake obsidian can bring
purity to mind and body and
help you see the light in dark-
ness. It is a wonderful healing
stone for times of transition and
stress and can aid you in finding
the lessons and gifts in hard times. Snowflake obsidian helps
to transmute denser energies into lighter frequencies and
gives you strength in moments of doubt.**

COLOR: Jet-black with white inclusions

ORIGIN: Argentina, Italy, Scotland, United States

ENERGY: Anchors, transmutes, integrates

CHAKRAS: Root, Crown

PAIRS WITH: Apophyllite, black tourmaline, clear quartz, Herkimer diamond, pyrite, Shungite, smoky quartz

SPECIAL CARE: Needs to cleansed often, as it absorbs and transmutes a lot of its surrounding energy.

Obsidian is an amorphous stone; unlike most minerals, its structure is not formed in any sort of geometric patterning. It is found in places of either past or present volcanic activity. Because it forms hard, sharp edges when broken, it has been used since prehistoric times to make tools, knives, and arrowheads.

Sunstone

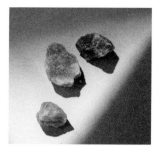

With a warming energy that radiates energy and life force, sunstone helps you trust your internal guidance and keep a positive disposition in all situations. It strengthens your intuition and helps you to step forward with determination and put your intuitive insights into motion. Work with sunstone to elevate the emotional body and cope with anxiety, seasonal affective disorder, and bouts of depression.

COLOR: Light orange to red, brown

ORIGIN: Canada, India, Russia, United States

ENERGY: Radiates, directs, activates

CHAKRAS: Solar Plexus, Crown, Sacral

PAIRS WITH: Amber, calcite, carnelian, citrine, clear quartz, Lemurian seed, pyrite

The name "sunstone" reflects the stone's coloration and warm sparkling inclusions, but it is also known as *aventurine feldspar*. Sunstone has been found upon Vikings' ships, and it is thought it was used as a navigational tool upon the seas.

Tiger's Eye

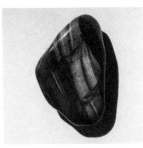

Tiger's eye is a grounding and strengthening stone. It helps to move energy internally within your body, which is in turn reflected in your external life. Tiger's eye stimulates your courage to pursue dreams and move forward with drive. Hematite inclusions help to ground the energy so that you may move forward on your path from a solid, grounded space. It helps activate and balance the Solar Plexus Chakra, anchoring your personal power in a place of integrity.

COLOR: Light brown to dark brown

ORIGIN: Australia, Burma, South Africa, United States

ENERGY: Magnetizes, amplifies, grounds

CHAKRAS: Root, Solar Plexus

PAIRS WITH: Amber, carnelian, citrine, hematite, Shungite, smoky quartz

Tiger's eye, a form of quartz, has an identifiable luster and silky appearance. Tiger's eye has been referred to as the "all-seeing, all-knowing eye" for allowing the wearer to see beyond the illusion of time and space. Roman soldiers who thought it held the energy of the sun would carry it into battle for courage and strength.

Turquoise

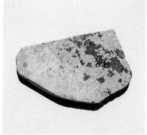

Long revered as a stone of protection, strength, healing, divination, and good luck, turquoise attunes you to the convergence of everything in the universe so that you may see yourself as the bridge between heaven and earth. Turquoise allows you to find balance between dark and light, earth and sky, and masculine and feminine energies. The healing and protective stone reminds you of the interconnections between all things and helps you see the sacred in everyday life.

COLORS: Light blue, blue-green, teal, brown

ORIGIN: Afghanistan, Australia, Iran, Tibet, United States (Southwest)

ENERGY: Amplifies, aligns, balances

CHAKRAS: Heart, Throat, Root

PAIRS WITH: Aventurine, calcite, chrysocolla, hematite, kyanite, moldavite, tiger's eye

Turquoise, a copper aluminum phosphate, is one of the most widely used and longest recorded gemstones, including Mesopotamian beads that date back to 5000 BC and ancient Chinese and Egyptian artifacts that are over 3,000 years old. Turquoise has been an important stone of the indigenous nations of the Americas, who have used it in ceremony and tribal exchange.

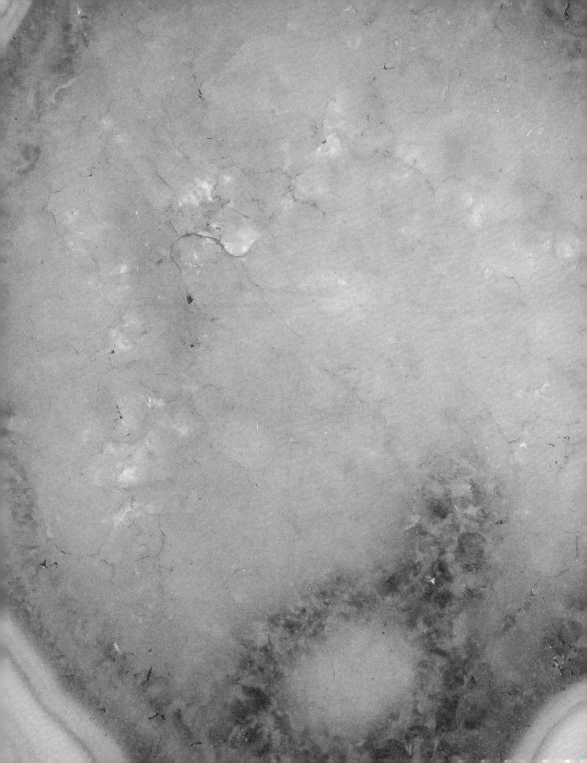

II

ENERGY,
STRENGTH,
and HEALING
RITUALS

SIX

For Wellness and Balance

WE CONTINUOUSLY TAKE IN INFORMATION ON A DAILY basis in the form of energy from the world around us. We then filter it through our own system and current level of awareness, subsequently experiencing thoughts, feelings, and emotions. It becomes imperative to stay present in what we are feeding our mind, body, and spirit, as it greatly affects our life. This chapter outlines daily energetic rituals that are key in sustaining long-term health and overall well-being.

149

DAILY ENERGETIC CLEANSE RITUAL

BEST TIME OF DAY: Morning or before bed
TIME NEEDED: 5 minutes
FREQUENCY: Daily or as frequently as needed
WHAT YOU'LL NEED: Selenite wand

This wellness ritual serves as an everyday energetic tune-up. Just as you brush your teeth daily for personal hygiene, you should maintain an energetic hygiene practice to sustain your overall vitality and well-being. When performed regularly, it will help cleanse daily energetic buildup and will allow you to tune in deeper to your own energetic fluctuations and strengthen the healer within you.

1 Hold the selenite wand in your right hand. Close your eyes and take several deep breaths, beginning to calm your mind and body. Allow your breath to soften any tension.

2 Set the intention to clear your energetic field of any unnecessary energetic residue from the day and to fill your body with healing light energy.

3 Use the selenite wand to cleanse your auric field by gently outlining the shape of your body, about 6 inches away from your skin. Begin by outlining your upper body, then move down your back, legs, and feet.

4 Once you've outlined your entire body, hold the selenite in both hands in front of your chest, aligning it vertically with your body.

5 Visualize breathing the energy of the selenite into your body, allowing the high frequency of the stone to cleanse and revitalize all of your cells.

6 Take a few deep breaths, and when you are ready, gently open your eyes.

REMOVING NEGATIVITY RITUAL

BEST TIME OF DAY: Night

TIME NEEDED: 10 minutes

FREQUENCY: Twice per month or as frequently as needed

WHAT YOU'LL NEED: Black tourmaline, selenite,
and sage leaves or Palo Santo

There are times in your life when things might simply seem "off." You may feel drained of energy or unwell. Perhaps you are unable to shake thoughts of worry or fear throughout the day. Or maybe the feeling is a result of frustrating or exhausting interactions with an individual, such as a coworker. As you traverse your daily life, you will come in contact with different energies and frequencies, including negative ones. As moths to a flame, dense energies attach to our light bodies, making us feel off. You don't need to fear these energy forms—instead, allow yourself to find a neutral space and simply cleanse your field of them.

1   Cleanse your immediate space and body with sage or Palo Santo.

2   Place the black tourmaline on the ground. With your feet hip width apart, stand over the black tourmaline. Hold the selenite in your right hand.

3   Say out loud:

"I choose to release all that no longer serves my highest purpose. Any residual energy that is not mine easily leaves my space now."

4   Close your eyes and deepen your breath.

continued…

151

For Wellness and Balance

5 Visualize any stuck or dense energy within your body gently releasing out the soles of your feet into the black tourmaline. Imagine any destructive habits, fearful thoughts, or dense influences in your life are swept to the black tourmaline and instantly transmuted.

6 You might feel a weight lifted within or your body simply becoming "lighter."

7 When you feel complete, say out loud:

"I consciously choose to call in only that which is supportive, loving, benevolent, and helpful in my life for my highest good.

I choose the light.

I choose the light.

I choose the light.

I rise above.

I rise above.

I rise above.

And so it is."

8 Take a deep breath and gently open your eyes.

9 After the ritual, sage the black tourmaline and place it in a bowl with sea salt for 1 to 2 hours to cleanse completely.

House Grid for Protection and Removing Negativity

To protect and remove negativity from your home, place a little pinch of salt in each corner of the house (not each room but each corner of the entire house). Then place a Shungite, black tourmaline, or black onyx in the corner. You may also place selenite wands alongside the walls of the house or under windowsills for added protection and potency.

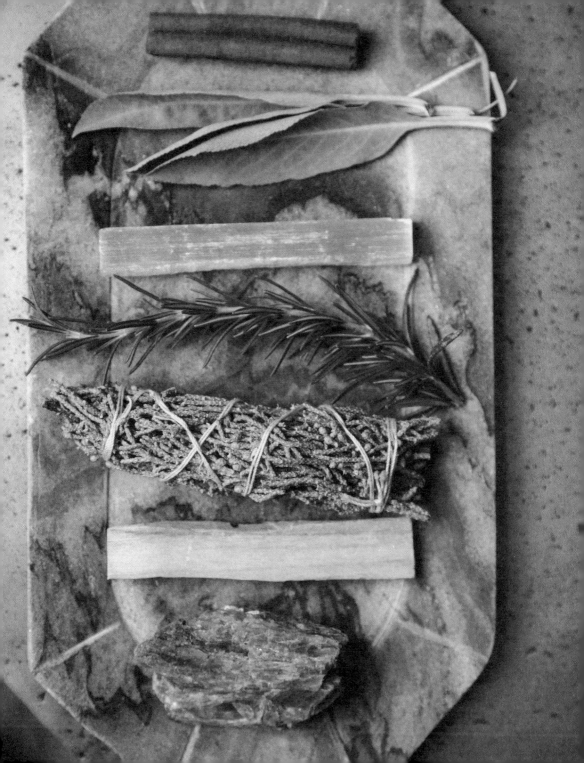

RELEASING PAIN RITUAL

BEST TIME OF DAY: Anytime
TIME NEEDED: 10 minutes
FREQUENCY: As frequently as needed
WHAT YOU'LL NEED: Amber, angelite, aragonite,
lepidolite, and raw emerald

This ritual creates a crystal grid on the body, which amplifies the healing energy of the crystals and directs it toward an area of physical inflammation and pain.

1 Lie down and get comfortable.

2 Place the amber on the area where you feel pain.

3 Hold the angelite in your right hand and the aragonite in your left hand. Rest the lepidolite on your chest or stomach, and place the emerald on your chest or center of heart. Allow the lepidolite to begin to soothe your nervous system as you close your eyes and start to deepen your breath.

4 Continue slow, deep breathing, counting 1-2-3-4 on your inhale and 5-4-3-2-1 on your exhale.

5 Now bring your awareness to the amber resting on the area. As you continue deep breathing, visualize the healing energy radiating into this area of discomfort, softening the pain, and sending information to the cells to regenerate and heal. Imagine with each deep exhale that the pain is softening and releasing.

6 Focus on your breath and allow the energy of the crystals to gently heal and recalibrate the place of pain. Repeat as needed.

7 Remain in this moment for a few minutes. Take a deep breath and gently open your eyes.

8 Remove the crystals from your body and cleanse the amber after the ritual.

BALANCING EMOTIONS RITUAL

BEST TIME OF DAY: Afternoon or evening
TIME NEEDED: 15 minutes
FREQUENCY: As frequently as needed
WHAT YOU'LL NEED: Lepidolite and smoky quartz

Emotions can be incredible indicators of how we are currently operating and what is being triggered in the moment, yet it is not always best to allow our emotions to run the show. This ritual helps to bring your emotional body into a place of balance, anchoring you into the present moment and enabling an energetic harmonization to occur within.

1   Find a comfortable seated position.

2   Place the lepidolite in your left hand and the smoky quartz in your right hand. Close your eyes.

3   Take a few deep breaths, and visualize the energy of the lepidolite making a semicircle in front of your body toward the smoky quartz. At the same time, the energy of the smoky quartz makes a semicircle around the back of your body toward the lepidolite. This creates a circular energy flow around you. Stay here for a few moments, letting the crystal energy build.

4   Visualize the circle of energy spiraling up around your body from your waist, until it reaches the top of your head. This energy then moves back down your body, reaching your feet.

5   Repeat this pattern at least three times. Each time, feel yourself bathed in the soothing and balancing light of the crystals.

6   When you feel grounded and peaceful, take a few deep breaths and open your eyes.

DETOX BATH RITUAL

BEST TIME OF DAY: Evening
TIME NEEDED: 30 minutes
FREQUENCY: 1 to 2 times per week
WHAT YOU'LL NEED: Smoky quartz, tumbled malachite,
½ cup baking soda, 1 cup Epsom salts, sage leaves,
rosemary sprigs, and sacred smoke or selenite

Just like a sponge that needs to be wrung out, your physical and ener-getic bodies need deep release from time to time. By slowing down, limiting time on electronics, spending more time in nature, eating simple home-cooked meals, drinking more water, getting ample sleep, and taking detox baths, you can help support your natural detoxifica-tion process and cleanse your mind, body, and spirit.

1 Set the intention to cleanse and release any disharmoni-ous energy from your body or energy field.

2 Fill the bath as hot as you can tolerate. Pour in Epsom salts and baking soda, then add sage leaves and rosemary sprigs.

3 Place the smoky quartz and malachite in the bathtub.

4 Get in the tub and gently close your eyes. Visualize any heavy energy releasing from your body and absorbing into the bathwater.

5 Remain in your heart, grate-ful for the minerals and herbs cleansing your body and restoring balance. Stay here for 30 minutes or until you break a light sweat. Gently open your eyes and take a few deep breaths.

6 Take the stones out of the bath, let the water drain, quickly rinse your body off, and step out of the bath.

7 Cleanse the healing crystals with sacred smoke or a sel-enite stone.

8 Notice how fresh and vibrant you feel.

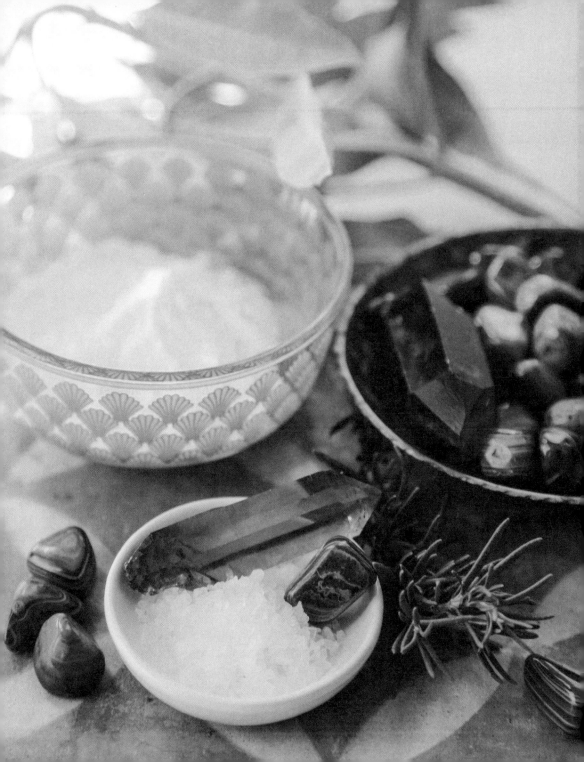

STRENGTHENING YOUR IMMUNITY RITUAL

BEST TIME OF DAY: Anytime
TIME NEEDED: 20 minutes
FREQUENCY: As frequently as needed
WHAT YOU'LL NEED: Amber, chrysocolla,
jadeite, ruby, and smoky quartz

A healthy immune system helps you stay strong in the face of modern assailants. This ritual brings you into full awareness of your body to help boost your immune system and encourage overall well-being and vibrancy. It's best to perform this ritual once per month, or more frequently to boost immunity during cold and flu season.

1 Lie down on your back in a comfortable area.

2 Place the ruby on your dantian, an energy center recognized by traditional Chinese medicine, which is 3 inches below your belly button. Place the amber on your thymus gland in the center of your chest and the chrysocolla on your thyroid by the center of your collarbone. Hold the jadeite in your right hand and the smoky quartz in your left hand.

3 Close your eyes and take three deep breaths. Bring your awareness to your right big toe and visualize and feel (if you can) the millions of cells vibrating within your big toe. Thank the cells in your toes for working to help you walk and move. Repeat this with your left big toe.

4 Repeat with your ankles, shins, knees, thighs, hips, glutes, and sexual organs, working your way up your body. Each time you bring your awareness to a new part of your body, say thank you, and visualize the cells in this area sparkling vibrantly.

5 Bring your awareness to your dantian, your wellspring of qi, or the current of energy within

the body and the measure of your vitality. Imagine breathing directly into your dantian, with the energy of the ruby penetrating deep into your cells.

6 Envision a ball of light in this area expanding and glowing with each inhale. On every exhale, you release waste and illness from your body. Breathe in and out 10 times, then continue up your body to your abdomen, upper abdomen, and breasts—acknowledging, sending gratitude, and seeing their cells filled with light.

7 Come to your thymus gland where the amber is resting. Visualize the warmth of the amber radiating deep into your thymus gland, pumping rays of light from this gland to your entire lymphatic system. Continue for 10 breaths.

8 Bring your awareness to your thyroid gland where you placed the chrysocolla. (If your thyroid has been taken out, you may still visualize its energy.) Breathe into the thyroid, and imagine the chrysocolla weaving its energy, gently balancing the thyroid, and releasing anything no longer needed. Fill your thyroid area with light, and see the light within the gland spread to your whole body.

9 Continue moving up to your lips, face, eyes, ears, until you reach the top of your head.

10 Once you reach the top of your head, visualize your entire body filled with light. Each cell is radiating pure vitality and light. Each system is in balance.

11 Say out loud:

"My body is in perfect harmony.

I am full of vitality.

My immune system is in balance.

I am strong, protected, supported.

I radiate vibrant light in all directions."

12 Remain here for as long as you wish. Then, take a few deep breaths, and bring yourself fully back into the present moment. Gently open your eyes.

SEVEN

The Power of Love

LOVE IS WHAT YOU ARE. IT IS THE ESSENCE OF THE VERY cells in your body and each strand of hair upon your head. You are love. And the power of love is stronger than any other frequency in the Universe. Love heals, love holds, love creates, love connects, love is all there is. It's the purest and most potent medicine. The rituals and minerals in this chapter connect you to the healing power of radical transformation through love.

SELF-LOVE RITUAL

BEST TIME OF DAY: Morning or night, ideally after bathing
TIME NEEDED: 10 to 30 minutes
FREQUENCY: Weekly, daily, or as frequently as needed
WHAT YOU'LL NEED: Rose quartz and Self-Love Oil

Truly everything comes back to self-love. The love you are able to give yourself is mirrored in the love you receive. It is a constant cosmic exchange. When you practice self-love, you remember that you are already perfect exactly as you are. You are, after all, pure love; there just might have been some things along the way that caused you to forget the divine perfection that is YOU! So go ahead, fall madly in love with yourself. Because you are amazing.

1   Prepare your Self-Love Oil and then take a bath.

2   After bathing, massage the oil into your body and repeat, "I love you" to each body part. For example, "I love you, legs. Thank you for helping me move." Keep thanking your body until you've massaged and expressed love to your whole body.

3   Place your hands on your heart and say out loud or to yourself:

    "I love you. I am here.

    I love you. I am here.

    I love you. I am here."

4   Feel the warmth of that love and the rose quartz radiating and circulating all around your body.

Self-Love Oil

INGREDIENTS:

¾ cup jojoba oil
(or another carrier
oil of your choice)

4 drops rose absolute
essential oil

3 drops jasmine
essential oil

2 oz. dried rose petals

Rose quartz

TOOLS/EQUIPMENT:

8 oz. glass jar

Dropper

1   Set your intention of self-love into the rose quartz by placing your hands over the crystal and saying:

"I embrace and love all that I am.

I am love. I am love. I am pure radiant love.

And I am incredible!"

2   Place the rose quartz in the jar, and pour the jojoba oil on top.

3   Using a dropper, add both jasmine and rose essential oil. Add the dried flowers. Cover the jar and swirl lightly.

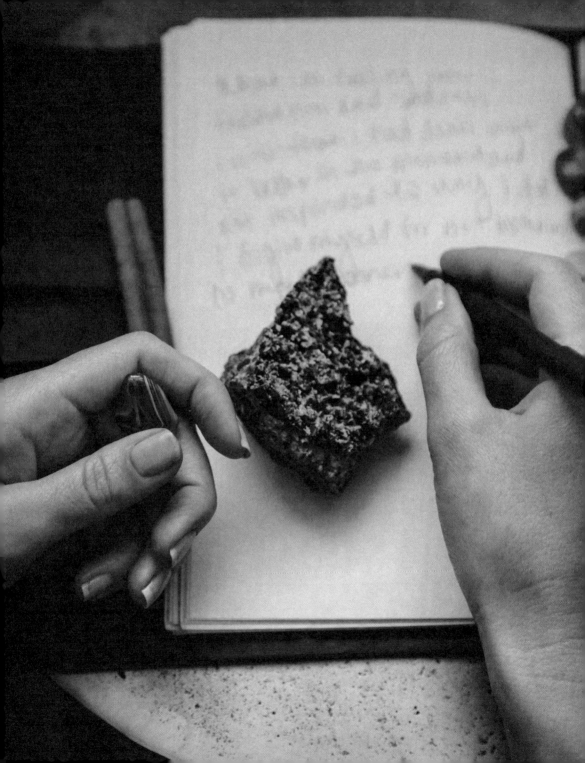

HELP WITH HEARTBREAK RITUAL

BEST TIME OF DAY: Anytime
TIME NEEDED: 30 minutes
FREQUENCY: As frequently as needed
WHAT YOU'LL NEED: Small tumbled malachite, ruby
fuchsite, pen, paper, and cinnamon stick

*Whether it is a romantic heartbreak, loss of a loved one, or friendship
breakup, our hearts hold the memories and wounds of these traumas.
But the beautiful thing is the heart is a muscle, and just like every other
muscle fiber that tears and rebuilds itself, the heart will heal and your
levels of love will be that much deeper. Perform this ritual to release old
energy and emotions and create space for new love to come in.*

1 Energetically cleanse yourself
with a cinnamon stick. Find a
seated position, and hold the
malachite in your hand.

2 Bring your awareness into your
heart, close your eyes, and
take a few deep breaths. Allow
yourself to tune into everything
you are currently feeling and
all that your heart is holding on
to. Gently open your eyes.

3 Write down the answers to these
prompts. Freewrite, or write the
first things that come to you.

What I'm feeling now is:

*How I wish this experience
had gone:*

I forgive myself for:

I love myself for:

This experience taught me:

The gift I received:

*I know in my heart of hearts
that one day:*

4 After you feel complete, you
may safely burn this paper or
shred it and bury it outside.
If you choose to bury it, plant
flowers or seeds over the
shredded paper.

5 Carry the ruby fuchsite with
you for at least 10 to 21 days
after performing this ritual.

ATTRACTING ROMANTIC LOVE RITUAL

BEST TIME OF DAY: Morning or night
TIME NEEDED: 20 minutes
FREQUENCY: Daily
WHAT YOU'LL NEED: Aventurine, rose quartz,
rose water, paper, and pen

This ritual helps to open your heart and magnetize your energetic field to attract a romantic partner. I performed this ritual daily (sometimes twice a day) for 30 days before meeting my husband years ago. It helped me get laser-focused and acclimate to the feeling I wanted to feel in my relationship, and when I eventually met him, I felt the exact feeling I had been meditating on for a month! Allow yourself to move beyond what your "list" is, and instead focus on how you want to feel. The perfect partner may come in an unexpected package! Try and remain neutral, open, and as patient as possible.

1   Spritz rose water on your heart and face. Sit down and find a comfortable position.

2   Close your eyes and connect to your heart. Tune into the partner you wish to call in. Think of the attributes and qualities they emanate and how they make you feel.

3   Tune into the feeling of what this romantic partnership feels like. Stay here for a few moments.

4   Open your eyes and write down on a piece of paper what qualities they hold and how you want to feel in this relationship.

5   Sit with the list in front of you. Place the rose quartz in your left hand and the aventurine in your right hand. These energies balance and open the Heart Chakra, emanating the balanced masculine and feminine energies within you and the balanced masculine

and feminine energies you wish to call in with this new love. (Remember, we all have masculine and feminine energies within us, regardless of our gender identities or sexual orientations.)

6   Bring your palms out in front of you as if someone is giving you a gift. Tune into the energies on the paper and the feeling of this new relationship. Hold this feeling within you.

7   Now bend your elbows and bring your hands to your heart and extend them back out. Repeat this multiple times, extending out to receive and draw into your heart as if your heart has an open door and you are welcoming this new energy of this relationship into your heart and into your life.

8   Keep holding the vision and the feeling, welcoming it into your heart.

9   You may say out loud or to yourself:

    "I welcome you into my life and into my heart."

10 Hold the vision and repeat this action for 5 to 10 minutes. (When you first begin your ritual practice, you may want to start with 5 minutes, then work your way up to 10 as you become more accustomed to it.)

11 Repeat the ritual every day for at least 30 days. Keep the rose quartz and aventurine by your bedside table or on your altar at night.

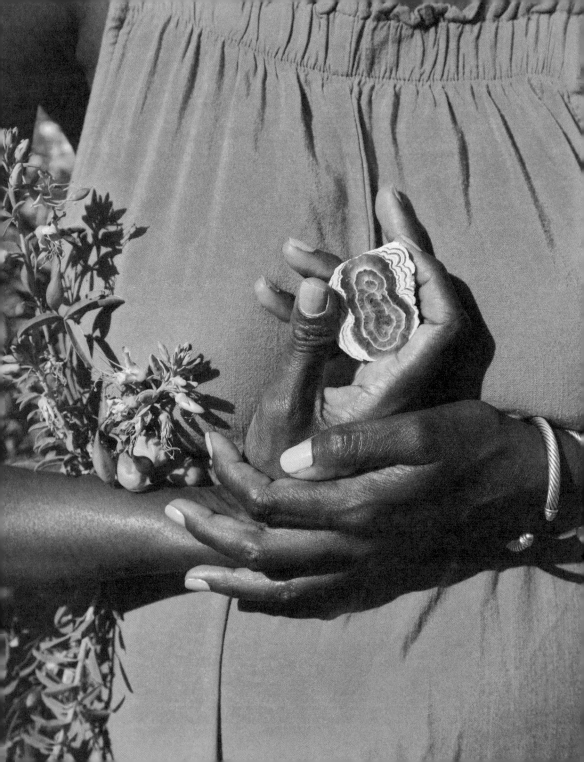

UNCONDITIONAL LOVE RITUAL

TIME OF DAY: Anytime
TIME NEEDED: 10 to 15 minutes
FREQUENCY: Weekly, daily, or as frequently as needed
WHAT YOU'LL NEED: Rhodochrosite

Unconditional love is the natural energy of the Universe; it is our home frequency. This type of love knows no boundaries, gender, or sexual orientation. It does not judge or control. It is the energy of oneness that connects everything together. When you vibrate at the frequency of unconditional love, you are in harmony with all of the world and all of creation.

1 Find a seated position and hold the rhodochrosite with both hands to your Heart Chakra in the center of your chest.

2 Close your eyes and deepen your breath. Connect to your heart, and imagine a pink magenta light glowing and radiating from it. This is a light of unconditional love. It holds only pure light, no attachments, and only full exchange of giving/receiving love.

3 Visualize your pink glowing orb in your heart, sending a line of pink magenta light to everyone in your household, including your pets. Now imagine this pure loving light reaching out to your extended family, friends, community, neighborhood, work, city, and state, and all across the country. Now imagine this magenta ray of light uniting everyone's hearts around the globe in pure unconditional love.

continued…

4   Extend the light to all the plants, to all the trees, flowers, and shrubs. To all the birds, insects, animals, and sea creatures. Imagine a whole web of magenta pink light radiating and connecting the whole world. Allow yourself to feel this unity, this oneness, this love.

5   Say out loud:

"I am love. I am love. I am love.

You are love. You are love. You are love.

All is love. All is love. All is love.

I spread love everywhere I go."

6   Feel this energy of oneness and natural unconditional love radiating out from all of your cells. Take a few minutes to truly anchor this feeling into your body.

7   Take a deep breath, feel your feet on the earth, and open your eyes.

8   Place the rhodochrosite by plants in your house or a communal area in your home to hold and radiate the healing energy of unconditional love.

OPENING YOUR HEART RITUAL

BEST TIME OF DAY: Anytime
TIME NEEDED: 15 minutes
FREQUENCY: Weekly, daily, or as frequently as needed
WHAT YOU'LL NEED: Kunzite and rose water

Our heart is the seat of the soul. An open heart connects us to all beings, allows for deepening relationships, makes space for new relationships, and strengthens our relationship within, the most important relationship of all. Opening your heart can make you feel at one with everyone and everything in the Universe; it can feel euphoric. But there may be times when opening your heart releases old wounds or traumas. This is okay! As the saying goes, we feel as we heal.

1   Spritz yourself with rose water and find a comfortable position.

2   Bring the kunzite to your heart and close your eyes.

3   Say out loud:

    "I am safe to soften. I gently open my heart."

4   Imagine with each breath that your heart begins to gently open, as if it is a rose, with each breath opening the petals gracefully to full bloom.

5   Notice how it feels to soften and open your heart. Does it feel good? Is it vulnerable or uncomfortable? Without judging, just notice. Remind yourself that you are safe and you are held.

6   Keep breathing into your heart for 5 to 10 minutes, then gently open your eyes.

7   When you finish, you may place the kunzite on your altar and place fresh flowers next to it, holding the energy of unconditional love.

The Power of Love

FORGIVENESS RITUAL

BEST TIME OF DAY: Night
TIME NEEDED: 30 minutes
FREQUENCY: As frequently as needed
WHAT YOU'LL NEED: Pink tourmaline, pen, and paper

The energy of forgiveness is nothing short of transformational. When you allow judgment, shame, anger, and feelings of betrayal and hurt to be absolved into love and compassion, it frees your heart and energy field of these wounds, as well as all others involved. Forgiveness is a revolutionary act of compassion, courage, and unconditional love. The energy of pink tourmaline helps to release pain in the heart while maintaining a softness and strength. Perform this ritual inspired by the Hawaiian Ho'oponopono prayer for reconciliation, to help open your heart into a space of healing forgiveness.

1 Spritz yourself with rose water.

2 Find a comfortable place to lie down.

3 Place the pink tourmaline on your heart.

4 Close your eyes and take three deep breaths.

5 Say out loud:

   "I let go. I let go. I let go.

   I love you. I love you. I love you.

   I'm sorry. I'm sorry. I'm sorry.

   I forgive you. I forgive you. I forgive you.

   Please forgive me. Please forgive me. Please forgive me.

   Thank you. Thank you. Thank you."

6 Take out your pen and paper and write a letter to whomever you are forgiving. It may even be a letter to yourself! Let yourself say everything you've wanted to say, everything you feel or felt, and anything else

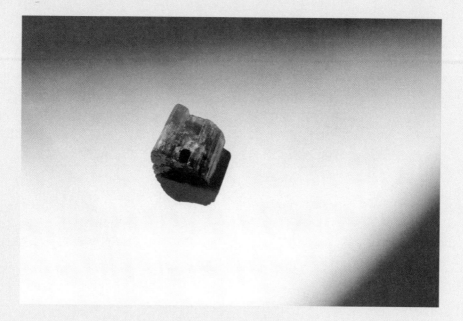

you wish to add. When your letter feels complete, fold the paper into four quadrants.

7   Say out loud:

"I let go. I let go. I let go.

I love you. I love you. I love you.

I'm sorry. I'm sorry. I'm sorry.

I forgive you. I forgive you.
I forgive you.

Please forgive me. Please forgive me. Please forgive me.

Thank you. Thank you.
Thank you."

8   You may safely burn the paper in a fireplace or fire pit, bury it in the earth, or shred it. Allow the energy to dissolve into love and transform in your heart.

EIGHT

Path to Finding You

T HE JOURNEY OF HEALING IS ULTIMATELY THE PROCESS OF remembering the truth of who you are. It may not always be easy, but it is always worth it. Luckily, you have an internal guidance system to help along your path. The minerals and rituals in this chapter are designed to activate your innate intuitive gifts and awaken you to your multidimensional creator-self.

175

BRINGING YOURSELF INTO ALIGNMENT RITUAL

BEST TIME OF DAY: Morning or night
TIME NEEDED: 20 minutes
FREQUENCY: 2 to 4 times per month, or as frequently as needed
WHAT YOU'LL NEED: Four clear quartz points, blue kyanite,
sage leaf or cinnamon stick, notebook, and pen

This ritual realigns your mind, body, and spirit; connects you to your highest path; and helps you to gain clarity on necessary actions needed for holistic well-being. Practice this ritual whenever you feel confused, lost along your personal path, fatigued, or overwhelmed. Repeat 2 to 4 times per month, daily, or as needed in times of stress. In this ritual, the clear quartz acts as an amplifier directing the energy toward you, and the kyanite aligns and rebalances your entire system.

1   Energetically cleanse yourself with a sage leaf or cinnamon stick.

2   Place the four clear quartz points in front, behind, and to the left and right of you. You want the point of the crystal toward you so that it directs and amplifies the energy toward you, not away.

3   Comfortably sit in the middle of the clear quartz crystals. Hold the kyanite in your lap.

4   Close your eyes and take three deep breaths. On each exhale, consciously release stress, worry, anxiety, and any dense energy from your body. Imagine this energy releasing down your body, out the soles of your feet, and into the earth.

5   Now visualize your body sur-
    rounded by a column of white
    light, a brilliant, nourishing
    golden light. The light extends
    all the way up into the cosmos,
    around and through your body,
    and down into the center of
    Earth. Remain in this column
    of light for several minutes,
    allowing your body to receive
    the light of the cosmos and the
    love of Earth.

6   In this open space, ask your
    Highest Self for guidance on
    any tangible steps you can
    take to move forward on your
    path in your highest align-
    ment. Stay open to what comes
    through, knowing if you do not
    receive an answer now, it will
    be revealed in the near future.
    Trust the timing.

7   Remain here in this activated
    light column for as long as you
    wish. When you feel complete,
    gently open your eyes and
    write down in your notebook
    any information that came
    through.

8   Close your notebook and
    repeat the following mantra
    three times:

    *"All is in alignment for my
    highest good. I choose to align
    with my highest potential."*

9   Close your eyes and allow
    the mantra to settle within
    your body and energetic field.
    Take a deep breath and open
    your eyes.

CONNECTING TO YOUR CREATIVE POTENTIAL RITUAL

BEST TIME OF DAY: Morning or afternoon
TIME NEEDED: 15 to 20 minutes
FREQUENCY: Weekly, daily, or as frequently as needed
WHAT YOU'LL NEED: Carnelian, kunzite, moonstone, and candle

You hold within you unlimited creative potential. This ritual connects you to the eternal Shakti energy within, the creative power of the Universe. Perform the activating ritual before embarking upon creative sessions, work, or conscious conception, or when you are feeling stuck, uninspired, or apathetic about your creativity. Let it light the fire within you, and let your creativity fuel and manifest your greatest dreams. This ritual is best performed during the day, as it is quite activating; however, try to find a space where you can create a darkened room so that you can focus on the candle.

1 Sit in a comfortable cross-legged position.

2 Place the carnelian in your lap (on your legs), the moonstone in your right hand, and the kunzite in your left hand with the candle in front of you.

3 Close your eyes and take some deep, centering breaths.

4 Open your eyes and light the candle. Take a few moments and gaze at the dancing flame. Notice the colors, feel the warmth, and witness the light created by this single flame. Invite the vision of the flame into your womb to reignite your own internal flame.

5   Envision the light of the flame flickering within your Sacral Chakra. Visualize a bright warm orange glow filling your womb. This is the spark of life, the spark of all creation. It glows brighter with each breath. The warmth radiates out from your womb and fills your entire body.

6   Say this activation mantra out loud:

"I am the flame that never goes out.

I create worlds upon worlds.

I birth life into form and visions into reality.

I fully embrace and activate my Divine Feminine Shakti, the powerful creatrix within, bringing forth new creations of endless possibility."

7   Feel your creative fire burning brightly, activating your divine creatrix within. This fire brings your creations into reality. Imagine and intend that this fire never burns out; it is a constant flame of creativity; it is ever burning.

8   Take a deep breath and open your eyes. Allow this energy to continue to move through you.

9   Try spending some time after this ritual to write, paint, sing, dance, or create in whatever way feels most inspiring.

179

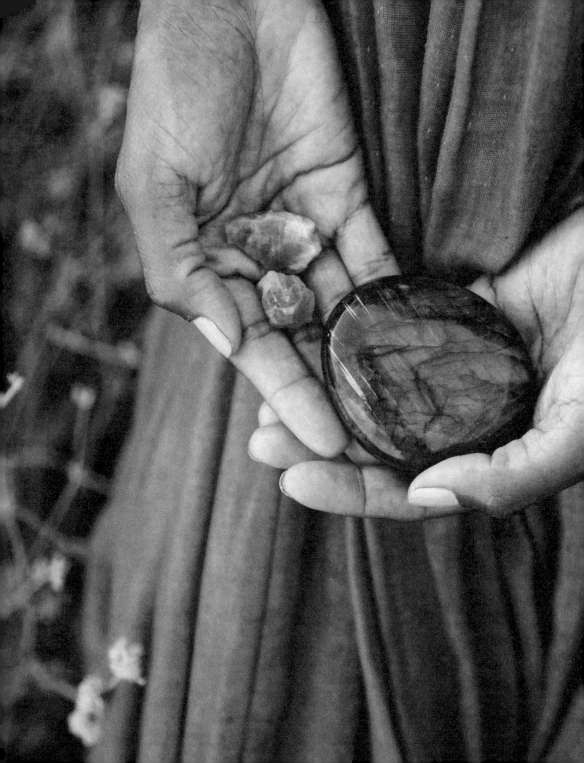

INNER REFLECTION AND REINVENTION RITUAL

BEST TIME OF DAY: Anytime
TIME NEEDED: 20 minutes
FREQUENCY: Seasonally, monthly, or as frequently needed
WHAT YOU'LL NEED: Labradorite and sunstone

When you live in a space of authenticity, in alignment with your own truth, and on your spiritual path, you will inevitably experience periods of transformation. Activities, foods, possibly even friendships that once brought you joy may stop resonating with you. It doesn't mean you won't ever again eat those foods or spend time with those individuals; it simply means your soul is calling you to experience something else. This ritual helps in times of change. It can be scary to reinvent yourself and not know what is on the other side, but trust that you are fully supported. The labradorite helps you access the new frequency you are stepping into, while the sunstone helps you take action in times of change.

1   Sit with the labradorite in your left hand and the sunstone in your right hand. Close your eyes and deepen your breath.

2   State out loud:

"I call upon my future self for support and assistance for my highest possible outcome."

3   Deepen your breath and visualize your future self 1 year from now. Your future self sits in front of you, smiling warmly, and is excited to see you and is supportive of your current transition.

continued…

4   What does she look like? What is she wearing? How does she feel? What does she smell like? Is she holding anything? Take note and feel her presence. Ask her:

How did you get to where you are now?

What steps can you take now on your journey?

5   Thank her for her support and guidance as she warmly blesses your sunstone and says she is available to support and help you every step of the way.

6   Say out loud or to yourself:

"I welcome new opportunity and expression of my highest self."

7   Take a moment to honor how far you've come and all you've faced and overcome to be who you are today. Place your hand on your heart and acknowledge the woman you are uncovering and all of the parts of yourself that are integrating and expanding.

8   Hold the vision of your future self in your mind's eye and imagine "imprinting" this vision into the sunstone.

9   Take a deep breath and open your eyes.

10 Carry the sunstone with you for 40 days.

RADIANT SELF-CONFIDENCE BATH RITUAL

BEST TIME OF DAY: Afternoon or evening
TIME NEEDED: 30 minutes
FREQUENCY: 1 to 2 times per week
WHAT YOU'LL NEED: Citrine, clear quartz, sunstone, lemon
balm, orange slices, and frankincense essential oil

*Allow yourself to be seen for the unique, bright light that you are! Perform
this ritual to activate and heal imbalances in the Sacral and Solar Plexus
Chakras, allowing you to embody the glowing goddess found within.*

1. Start the bathwater and place the orange slices and lemon balm in the water. Place the citrine, sunstone, and clear quartz into the water.

2. Outside the bathtub, close your eyes and take a deep breath. Anoint your Sacral, Solar Plexus, and Third-Eye Chakras with the frankincense oil diluted with a carrier oil.

3. Say out loud:

   *"I stand in my full power.
   I stand in my truth. I stand
   in my knowing."*

4. Open your eyes and get into the bath. Take several deep breaths. Allow the plants and crystals to brighten your energy field with their golden essence and weave their healing into your Sacral and Solar Plexus Chakras.

5. Close your eyes. Imagine yourself standing in one of your favorite places in the world. Envision yourself in full joyful expression as you radiate your pure essence.

6. Allow yourself to bathe in this healing frequency for 20 to 30 minutes. Hold the vision of you in your truest expression and anchor it into your Sacral and Solar Plexus Chakras.

7. Open your eyes and take several deep breaths. Slowly begin to bring yourself fully to the present moment.

SURRENDERING TO THE UNIVERSE RITUAL

BEST TIME OF DAY: Anytime
TIME NEEDED: 15 minutes
FREQUENCY: Weekly, daily, or as frequently as
needed, particularly in times of change
WHAT YOU'LL NEED: Clear quartz, lapis
lazuli, moldavite, and sage leaves

There are times when we are asked to practice deep trust and surrender all control to the Universe. Know and remember that everything is happening for you, not to you. Even if it is hard to see at the moment, trust in the divine orchestration that is underway. Your highest self, angels and guides, and the Universe are coconspiring for you, so now is the time to release fear, open your heart, and have faith in the Universe. You are always supported. This ritual is for when you are feeling lost, uncertain of next steps, or when things aren't going as you hoped. Allow this to align you into the vibration of openness and trust, staying aware of opportunities that may present themselves from the Universe.

1   Energetically cleanse yourself with sage. Find a place you can lie down. Set a timer for 15 minutes.

2   Place the clear quartz on your abdomen, the moldavite on your heart, and the lapis lazuli on your Third-Eye Chakra.

3   Allow the energies to begin to activate and attune. Take deep breaths to circulate vital life force through your body and move the crystalline energies deep within your cellular structure.

4   Repeat out loud three times:

"I awaken to my highest potential.

I surrender to the flow of the Universe.

I am in harmony with all of creation.

I release. I release. I release.

I allow. I allow. I allow.

I am free. I am free. I am free.

All the Universe is supporting me.

All the Universe is supporting me."

5   Close your eyes and remain here in meditation. Allow your energy to recalibrate, and stay open to any guidance that wishes to come through in the form of visions, images, words, memories, insights, or intuitive nudges. Practice staying neutral and open.

6   When your alarm goes off, gently deepen your breath and open your eyes. If you wish, write down any insights or guidance that came to you.

7   Repeat daily or weekly in times of change and transition.

AWAKENING YOUR INTUITION RITUAL

BEST TIME OF DAY: Anytime

TIME NEEDED: 10 minutes

FREQUENCY: Daily for 30 days, then as frequently as needed

WHAT YOU'LL NEED: Himalayan quartz, K2, and Opal

We are all born with an internal navigation system called intuition. It may be most familiar to you as a gut feeling. You may have trouble making sense of these internal nudges because intuition is like an instrument—it requires practice, patience, and trust to play. To reawaken your intuition and practice letting it flow, try performing this ritual daily for 30 days. If it's at first difficult to connect with your intuition, focus on simply noticing and staying present and neutral. With practice, you will learn to trust the information you receive, even if the answers sometimes surprise you.

1   Sit in a comfortable position on the floor with opal directly to your left, Himalayan quartz in your hands resting in your lap, and the K2 directly to your right.

2   Close your eyes and slow your breathing.

3   State internally to yourself:

"I awaken to my intuitive gifts within.

I choose to consciously listen to my intuition and trust my internal nudges.

I am always guided."

4   Stay in a space of quiet meditation for a few minutes.

5   Begin to ask yourself yes or no questions, big questions such as: Is it in my highest potential to accept this new job offer? Is it in my highest potential to go on this upcoming trip with my friends? Small questions can also help you tune

into your intuition: Is it in my highest interest to watch this extra episode of TV tonight? Do I need to go for a run? Do I need to take a nap? Begin with just three to five questions. Allow 30 seconds to 1 minute between each question.

6   Observe how your internal body feels when you state the words and ask the question. Notice if your body expands or contracts. It is a subtle sensation that takes practice tuning into. A *yes* sensation is expansive, and a *no* sensation is contractive.

7   Practice with a few questions for a few minutes in meditation. If you don't feel anything at first, stay present and neutral. Simply notice any emotions that may arise. If nothing arises after a minute, move on to the next question. The answers we receive from our intuition aren't always the easiest or most convenient, which is why our minds often ignore it. Simply allow yourself to stay present and neutral with the information you receive.

8   Open your eyes and take several deep breaths.

9   Carry these stones with you over the next few weeks. Continue to ask big and small questions to yourself throughout the day to strengthen this self-feedback muscle. Practice staying tuned into your intuitive nudges throughout the day.

NINE

Anxiety and Depression

A S YOU BECOME YOUR OWN HEALER, YOU STRENGTHEN
the ability to bring yourself into balance at any time.
In this age of technology and information overload, it
becomes of utmost importance to have practices and tools
that center, ground, and calm in times of need. The rituals
and crystals in this chapter help bring mindful awareness
and peace into your day during the times you need it most.

GROUNDING RITUAL

BEST TIME OF DAY: Morning or night
TIME NEEDED: 5 minutes
FREQUENCY: Weekly, daily, or as frequently needed
WHAT YOU'LL NEED: Garnet, hematite,
Kambaba jasper, and smoky quartz

Our modern days are so filled with emails, meetings, appointments, social commitments, and family responsibilities that it sometimes feels as though we can hardly catch our breath. This ritual is for anchoring and grounding your energy into your body, quieting the nervous system, and calling on the support of Mother Earth to strengthen your roots into the earth. Our grounding roots are invisible energetic ties to the earth, helping us stay connected and in harmony. Use this quick ritual when feeling anxious, overwhelmed, stressed, overburdened, or overworked.

1   Sit in a comfortable position on the floor or in a chair.

2   Create a crystal grid by placing the Kambaba jasper in front of you, garnet to your right, hematite behind you, and smoky quartz to your left. The sacred geometry will help anchor your energetic field and support grounding.

3   Close your eyes and begin to deepen your breath.

4   Bring your awareness to the base of your spine and into the ground beneath you. Imagine your spine extends down as roots growing through the floorboards of the building and into the different layers of the earth, all the way down until they reach the center of Earth. Imagine your roots anchoring into Earth's center.

5   Feel the support of the earth as gravity presses down and your roots sink in. Just like a plant draws water from the soil, allow your roots to drink up nourishing golden energy from the earth. Draw it back up into the base of your spine. Allow the grounding and nourishing earth energy to begin filling your body. It moves through your arms, fingers, shoulders, neck, face, ears, and top of your head.

6   Feel your whole body fill with the grounding energy of the earth. Set the intention that your grounding root stays anchored into the earth no matter where you go.

7   Say out loud or quietly to yourself three times:

*"I am safe. I am present.
I am connected. I am grounded.
I am here."*

8   Allow your breath to deepen. Feel yourself fully present in this moment, in your body, on Earth. Let this feeling settle within your body.

9   Take a deep breath and open your eyes. Repeat as often as needed throughout the day or week.

DAILY MINDFULNESS MEDITATION RITUAL

Meditation is a ritual of returning to oneself. It is a practice of slowing down, looking within, and finding home. Quieting the noise and turning inward a few moments every day can lessen anxiety and stress and help you hear the messages from your heart. Start with 5 minutes a day and increase the time slowly. Allow your meditation practice to be your daily recharge.

1   Place the amethyst in your lap or in the palm of your hand.

2   Find a comfortable position, sitting or lying down, and gently close your eyes. Allow your body to soften. Notice places within your body that may be holding tension or stress, and gently let it release.

3   Deepen your breath, letting your breath expand all the way down to your toes. Each breath fills your body completely, and you exhale all the way out. Keep your awareness on your breath.

4   Let each inhale and exhale bring you deeper into yourself. As thoughts or distractions arise, become aware of the thought, and bring yourself gently back to your breath.

5   Allow the amethyst to gently awaken your Third-Eye Chakra.

6   Remain in this place of deep breath awareness for 5 to 30 minutes.

7   When complete, gently open your eyes and bring your full presence back.

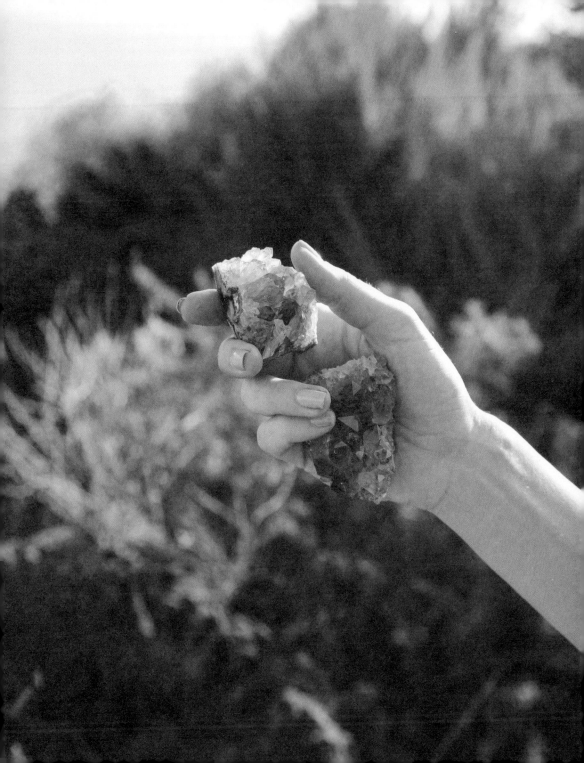

CALMING YOUR MIND RITUAL

BEST TIME OF DAY: Anytime
TIME NEEDED: 10 minutes
FREQUENCY: Daily or as frequently as needed
WHAT YOU'LL NEED: Howlite and Palo Santo or incense

*Nowadays, we take in so much information in a single day. It's easy
for our nervous system to become overwhelmed and our minds to race
a mile a minute. Meditation and mantra (japa) meditation can be
great to calm the mind and ease system overload. Allow the energy of
howlite and recite the following "ram" mantra to center and balance an
overactive mind. "Ram" brings you back to the infinite you within and
represents living each day in harmony.*

1 You may cleanse with Palo
   Santo beforehand or light an
   incense.

2 Sit in a comfortable position on
   the floor. Place the howlite in
   one palm, while the other hand
   rests palm side up.

3 Set an alarm for 10 minutes.
   Gently close your eyes and let
   your breath begin to deepen
   melodically and in a natural
   rhythm. Repeat "Let" on your
   inhale and "go" on your exhale
   three times.

4 Begin to recite the mantra "Ram, ram, ram, ram"

(pronounced "rāhm") silently
to yourself. You may go as
quickly or as slowly as you like.
Let the sound resonate and
reverberate within your being.
Feel your body begin to ground
as you continue to focus on
the mantra. As your mind
and small self begin to sink
into the expanse, fill yourself
with the nourishing energy of
this mantra.

5 When the alarm bell rings, take
   a deep breath and gently open
   your eyes.

IMPROVING SLEEP RITUAL

BEST TIME OF DAY: 1 to 2 hours before bedtime
TIME NEEDED: 20 minutes
FREQUENCY: Daily or as frequently as needed
WHAT YOU'LL NEED: Howlite, rose quartz, smoky quartz, selenite, and lavender essential oil

Healthy sleep habits are essential for overall holistic well-being. This ritual helps bring the body into a place of balance and peace, allowing you to release stress from the day and slip off into the dream world. Before you begin your ritual, consider turning off all screens and blue-light-emitting technology and keeping all electronics in airplane mode with Wi-Fi turned off.

1   Anoint your Third-Eye Chakra, in the middle of your forehead, with one drop of lavender essential oil diluted in a carrier oil, and rub any remaining oil into the soles of your feet.

2   Lie down and place the smoky quartz at your feet, the rose quartz on the middle of your chest, the howlite on your Third-Eye Chakra, and the selenite above your head.

3   Let go of any stress or anxieties from the day. Visualize them flowing from above your body, out your feet, and into the smoky quartz.

4   Visualize the soothing energy of the howlite and rose quartz radiating throughout your body, and envision the selenite pouring cleansing light energy down from the top of your head. Remain here for a few minutes.

5   When it is time to fall asleep, remove the smoky quartz and selenite. You may sleep with the rose quartz or howlite under your pillow for peaceful dreamtime.

BEST TIME OF DAY: Anytime

TIME NEEDED: 10 minutes

FREQUENCY: Daily or as frequently as needed

WHAT YOU'LL NEED: Lepidolite

Most days it can feel as if we're pulled in a million directions, and it can be overwhelming. Yet when we slow down, get grounded, and thus calm our nervous system, we can see clearly what needs to be attended to, what doesn't, and how we can best handle any given situation. The power stone in this ritual is lepidolite, a healing crystal that can facilitate instant stress relief.

1   Turn off your phone and Wi-Fi (if possible), and lie down on your back.

2   Place the lepidolite on your Third-Eye Chakra and close your eyes.

3   Let your body get heavy and feel as if you are melting into the floor. Invite the energy of lepidolite into your body and cells, allowing the natural lithium within the mineral to gently soothe and wash away any stress or anxieties.

4   Feel the lepidolite wash down your face, neck, arms, and fingers and move into your toes. Drop into the sensation of being bathed in the relaxing emanations of lepidolite.

5   Remain here for as long as you like. Let go of worry and doubt, and trust in the current of all that is.

6   Say out loud:

"I am in ease and flow with all of life. I easily let go. I am in rhythm with all that is."

7   Allow yourself to rest here for another few minutes, then take a deep breath and gently open your eyes.

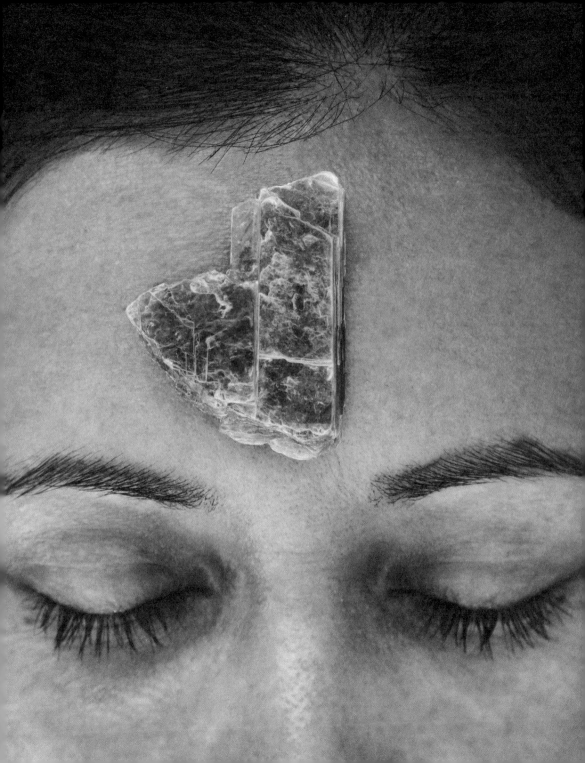

TEN

Fertility and Pregnancy

THE JOURNEY OF BRINGING FORTH CHILDREN INTO THIS modern world is as unique to each mother as the soul coming in. From conception to birth to postpartum, each step along the way brings new aspects of discovery and deeper layers of love and devotion. The rituals in this chapter create sacred containers and energetic activations along the path to motherhood.

199

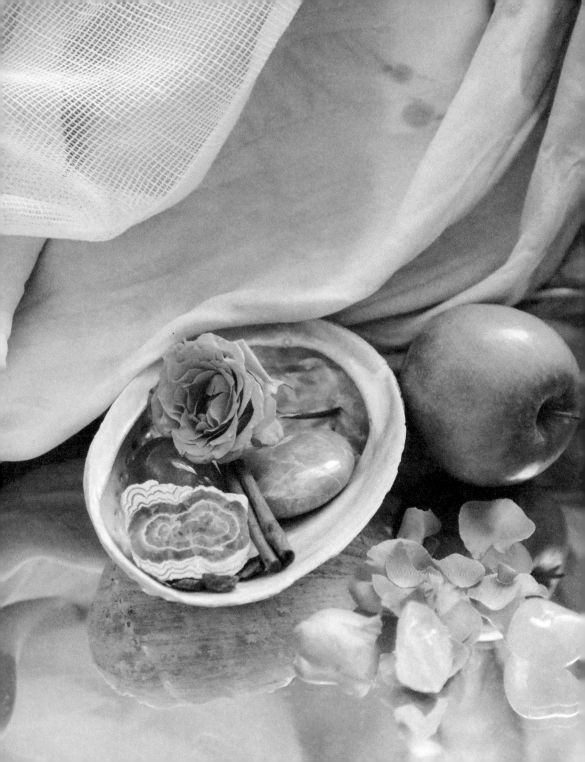

FERTILITY AND CONCEPTION RITUAL

BEST TIME OF DAY: Anytime
TIME NEEDED: 15 to 25 minutes
FREQUENCY: Weekly, daily, or as frequently as needed
WHAT YOU'LL NEED: Peach moonstone, raw ruby,
rhodochrosite, cinnamon stick, apple, and rose

This ritual connects you to your natural fertility and creates an energetic opening within your womb for conception. The rose, apple, and ruby have long been revered as symbols of the Divine Feminine and female fertility. Allow the energy of these sacred talismans and the healing crystals to strengthen your connection with your womb, and begin to tune into the energy of your spirit baby.

1   Energetically cleanse yourself with the cinnamon stick. Lie down, placing the rose and apple by your side.

2   Place the ruby on your Sacral Chakra/womb, the peach moonstone below your belly button, and the rhodochrosite on your heart.

3   Close your eyes and tune into your womb. Envision it as a glorious garden, filled with your favorite flowers, lush plants, and ripe fruit trees. There are butterflies and honey bees, and your womb garden is full of life and potential.

4   Visualize yourself in the garden, under the shade of an apple tree, with a child in your arms. Look into the eyes of the child and feel their breath against your skin and your heart overflowing with love for your child. There is an apple that is perfectly ripe next to you, and you bite into the juicy fruit, thanking the tree and nature for this blessing and gift.

5   Continue to envision your garden in fertile bloom, and take a moment to speak to your spirit baby if you feel called.

continued...

201

6   Say out loud:

"I honor the Divine Feminine within my womb full of life.

I am open to receive. I am ready to receive.

I trust the Divine Feminine within to create life within my fertile waters.

My body is a temple of divine love."

7   Allow yourself a few minutes to rest and integrate in this space. Take a deep breath and gently open your eyes.

8   Eat your blessed apple, and place the rose with crystals on your altar or next to your bedside.

MISCARRIAGE HEALING RITUAL

BEST TIME OF DAY: Night
TIME NEEDED: 5 to 10 minutes
FREQUENCY: Daily for 30 days
WHAT YOU'LL NEED: Black tourmaline, pink tourmaline, ruby fuchsite, and selenite

The loss of a pregnancy at any stage can be extremely difficult to process. This healing ritual helps your feelings surface for deeper processing and begin to trust your body once more. It is best performed when you feel ready to integrate your emotions and wish to become pregnant again. Remember that there is no right or wrong way to feel when coping with grief.

1 Using the selenite as a cleansing wand, gently cleanse your energy and body. (See "Daily Energetic Cleanse Ritual," p. 150.)

2 Lie down in a comfortable position. Place the black tourmaline at your feet, the pink tourmaline on your Sacral Chakra/womb, and the ruby fuchsite on your heart. You may place the selenite above your head or hold it in your hands.

3 Close your eyes, then take a few deep breaths and tune into your heart. Allow whatever emotions are present to rise to the surface.

4 Intend for the stones to facilitate a gentle release as you feel the emotions move through you.

203

continued…

5   Say out loud:

"*I honor the divine intelligence of my body.*

I trust and know my body can become pregnant again.

My body is working with me.

My body is working with me.

My body is working with me."

6   Place one hand on your womb and the other hand on your heart. Take three deep breaths. Say to yourself:

"*I love you. I love you. I love you.*"

7   Gently open your eyes and take a deep breath.

8   As these stones are facilitating deep healing throughout the month, cleanse the ruby fuchsite, pink tourmaline, and black tourmaline every few days.

LOVING CONNECTION AND CONCEPTION RITUAL

BEST TIME OF DAY: Anytime
TIME NEEDED: 30 minutes
FREQUENCY: As frequently as needed on days
leading up to and during ovulation
WHAT YOU'LL NEED: Carnelian, peach
moonstone, rose quartz, and ruby

This ritual weaves together the conscious and loving intention between partners for conception. It may be performed before intercourse, insemination, or implantation. The energy created in this ritual is activated by the Heart Chakras of both partners and is amplified by the healing crystals. It brings both partners into a state of open receptivity and connection with the soul of the child they wish to bring into the world. You may repeat your ritual and blessing each time before trying to conceive.

1   Sit face-to-face with your partner.

2   The partner who is conceiving the child places the ruby on her lap or body. The partner supporting or facilitating holds the carnelian in their hands.

3   Place the rose quartz on the ground between both partners. Hold the peach moonstone together.

4   Begin to deepen and lengthen your breath together. Look deep into each other's eyes and begin breathing in unison.

5   Close your eyes now and connect to your hearts. Imagine a stream of love flowing from your heart to your partner's heart. Then envision a stream of love flowing from your heart to your womb.

continued…

Fertility and Pregnancy

6   Say a prayer and intention out loud to the loving soul you wish to call in. Envision welcoming this being into your heart, your body, and your life. Stay open to receive.

7   Stay here with your partner for a few moments. Take a deep breath together as you both gently open your eyes.

8   Remain in this loving, receptive space for as long as you wish before conscious conception or implantation.

9   If you feel called, you may write down a prayer or write a letter to your child. Place the rose quartz and peach moonstone on top of your prayer or letter, and place the carnelian and ruby on either side of the paper. Place the prayer or letter on your altar or in a place where you can see it every day.

PREPARING FOR BIRTH RITUAL

BEST TIME OF DAY: Anytime
TIME NEEDED: 20 minutes
FREQUENCY: Once, at approximately 35 to 36 weeks of pregnancy
WHAT YOU'LL NEED: Amethyst, chrysocolla, Kambaba jasper, smoky quartz, unakite, lavender essential oil, frankincense essential oil, peppermint essential oil, essential oil diffuser, and carrier oil

Every birth is as different and unique as the individual soul entering the world. This ritual of blessing your birth crystals to have during childbirth can provide additional support during the process. It helps you to get clear on your birth plan and stay grounded and present amid any changes that arise. A few weeks prior to your due date, begin to collect items you wish to have with you in your birth space. Whether birthing in a hospital, birthing center, or at home, these items will help bring comfort, strength, and support during the process.

This ritual can be done privately at home by yourself, with your family members, or as part of a baby shower. The intention and magic of this ritual is to fill the stones with love and support to be carried into and held during birth.

1   Place your hands over the smoky quartz, unakite, amethyst, chrysocolla, and Kambaba jasper.

2   Close your eyes and connect to your heart. Connect to the strength, beauty, and power of all women who have come before you, women birthing children since the beginning of dawn. Ask that they bring you strength, fortitude, and love. Call upon your ancestors—the women on your maternal side and the women on your paternal side—that they may send wisdom, grace, and courage.

continued…

3   Now set your own intention into these stones so that they may radiate this intention and energy for you throughout your entire birth.

4   Place these stones in your birth bag, or set them aside for when the time comes.

5   Once you've settled into your birthing room or hospital room, hold the chrysocolla and unakite in your hand or place them near your body for support and pain relief. Place the smoky quartz near your feet, beneath your mattress or bed and the Kambaba jasper beneath your body, under the mattress, or directly under the bed. Place the amethyst on a bedside table nearby.

6   You may place a selenite in the windowsill if birthing in a hospital or birthing center. Just remember to grab all of your stones when you are ready to go home.

7   You can also anoint yourself with diluted frankincense essential oil when contractions start. Lavender, frankincense, and peppermint essential oil are also soothing to diffuse during labor.

WELCOMING NEW LIFE RITUAL

BEST TIME OF DAY: Anytime

TIME NEEDED: 5 to 10 minutes

FREQUENCY: Once on the day of birth or
within the baby's first few months

WHAT YOU'LL NEED: Celestite, peach moonstone, and sage leaf

What a joyous miracle and blessing it is to welcome new life into the world! This crystal blessing celebrates the moment this beautiful soul came to earth. It calls upon prayers of love and light for the child and allows the crystals to hold prayers, intentions, and blessings for the future. It can be performed by you, the mother, or a friend or family member. Celestite in this crystal blessing calls upon the celestial world and guardian angels to bless and protect the baby while peach moonstone creates a peaceful, loving environment in the nursery to welcome the baby.

1   Cleanse the celestite and peach moonstone with sacred smoke or herbs.

2   Hold both stones in your hands and connect to your heart, saying thank you for the arrival of this new soul into the world.

3   Put the celestite in your left hand and the peach moonstone in your right hand.

4   Say this prayer out loud:

"Thank you for bringing this beautiful soul into the world. May they be held by the moon, warmed by the sun, protected by the trees, and nourished by the waters. May they be forever wrapped in love's light, as angels watch over this being of pure light."

continued…

209

Fertility and Pregnancy

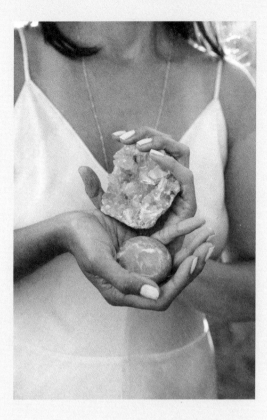

5 Visualize this prayer "imprinted" within the crystal lattice. You may say any additional prayers or loving intentions into the stone. Connect to gratitude in your heart for this new baby.

6 Place the stones in the nursery or whenever the baby sleeps.

Supportive Stones for the Nursery

Angelite	Lemurian Seed
Apophyllite	Lepidolite
Calcite	Peach Moonstone
Celestite	
Jade	Rose Quartz
	Scolecite

POSTPARTUM HEALING RITUAL

BEST TIME OF DAY: Anytime
TIME NEEDED: 5 minutes
FREQUENCY: As frequently as needed
WHAT YOU'LL NEED: Angelite, moss agate, and lavender essential oil

Congratulations! You made it through childbirth. This time isn't just about becoming a new mother—it's also about nurturing and mothering yourself. Traditionally, new mothers were surrounded by other women in their community who would help with cooking, cleaning, tending to the other children, dressing wounds, and making sitz baths, but that's not always the case anymore. Regardless of the support you have, look at this as a time to rest, recover, and heal.

1   Anoint the sides of your temples with lavender oil diluted with a carrier oil.

2   Lie down comfortably on your back. Place the angelite on your belly, and hold the moss agate in your hand. The angelite acts as an incredible healer and begins to help cool inflamed tissues and activate cellular regeneration.

3   Hold the moss agate and simply allow yourself to come into your heart. Close your eyes and take several deep breaths, bringing yourself to the present moment right now.

4   Say the following mantra out loud three times:

    "I am present. I am powerful. I am supported. I give myself permission to fully rest and heal."

5   Feel yourself in this present moment, in your body, with your feet on the ground.

6   Take a deep breath in, and gently open your eyes.

7   Carry the moss agate with you, and rub the stone anytime you need a reminder of this mantra.

ELEVEN

The Feminine Cycle

THE FEMININE ARCHETYPES WE EXPLORE AS WOMEN CAN be reflected in the cycles of our bodies. Regardless if we rear children or not, many women move through the Divine Feminine energies, presenting as Maiden, Mother, Enchantress, and Crone, which also correspond to menses, pregnancy/motherhood, and menopause. Ultimately, our relationship to the feminine cycle doesn't define us as women, but the rituals and crystals in this chapter can help connect you to your own internal feminine cycle as a way to awaken the Divine Feminine within.

EASING PMS RITUAL

BEST TIME OF DAY: Anytime
TIME NEEDED: 15 minutes
FREQUENCY: As frequently as needed in the 10 to
14 days leading up to menstrual cycle
WHAT YOU'LL NEED: Bloodstone, chrysocolla, ruby
fuchsite, and rose geranium essential oil

In ancient days, women were honored for their increased sensitivity and heightened intuition in the time leading up to menstruation, a time when suppressed emotions surface, allowing you to finally "speak your mind." Use ritual time to take inventory of what worked and what didn't over the past moon cycle as you prepare to release energetically and physically through your period.

1   Energetically cleanse yourself with a cinnamon stick or sage.

2   Lie down comfortably on your back. Place a drop of the rose geranium essential oil (diluted in a carrier oil) in the center of your womb, on your heart, and on your throat.

3   Place the bloodstone on your belly button, the chrysocolla over your right ovary, and the ruby fuchsite over your left ovary. You may rest your hands by your side or on your belly.

4   Repeat out loud:

"I trust my body, my watery currents within, aligning Earth's rhythm with mine.

A pure reflection of the moon, I open to the great mystery.

My depth and dreams come forth.

I let go of what is no longer needed and emerge anew."

5   Close your eyes and remain in this space for 5 minutes so that the stones can weave their vibration into your womb.

6   Take a deep breath and gently open your eyes.

Stones for PMS and Cramps

Amber	Jade
Angelite	Lepidolite
Aragonite	Moonstone
Carnelian	Rose Quartz
Chrysocolla	Ruby

PERIMENOPAUSE RITUAL

BEST TIME OF DAY: Anytime
TIME NEEDED: 15 to 20 minutes
FREQUENCY: As frequently as needed
WHAT YOU'LL NEED: Unakite and clary sage essential oil

Often referred to by women as "the Change," the transitional cycle of perimenopause is a transformational passage in your life. As your physical body goes through a major physical shift, deep internal changes also occur on an emotional, spiritual, and mental level. You might experience anxiety, anger, hormonal shifts, body temperature changes, and anything in between. Throughout perimenopause and into menopause, let this ritual ground you into the initiation you are embarking on, surrounded by legions of women who have traversed this path before, holding you and cheering you on. The passage and initiation into a new phase of life is to be celebrated and honored.

1 Anoint your womb with the clary sage essential oil (diluted in a carrier oil).

2 Lie down on your back and place the unakite on your womb, or sit down and hold it in your hand.

3 Close your eyes and let your breath gently expand and deepen.

4 Visualize yourself by a beautiful emerald-colored waterfall, surrounded by luscious plants and the scent of night-blooming jasmine. There is moisture in the air, but a cool breeze blows against your hair. You see an area with gorgeous blankets and tea set out for you, and you sit down. Your grandmothers appear and sit next to you. One puts a warm shawl over your shoulders, and

the other pours you tea. You notice there are many women here peeking out from the trees; they are here to support, celebrate, and honor you.

5 Allow yourself to be held in this moment. You tell your story to the women and tell them what you are currently experiencing in your life and this transition. They listen intently, and you can feel the love pouring out. They motion to the emerald pond, and you get up and enter the pool. The cool water cleanses your skin and refreshes your spirit.

6 You remember how supported you are in this web of life and the importance of this next phase of your journey. The water releases stagnant energy and leaves you feeling vibrant. You thank the women and your grandmothers, and they ask that you return here whenever you wish. You take one more inhale of the sweet night-blooming jasmine. On your exhale, you open your eyes and are back in your space.

7 Carry this unakite in your pocket or purse for the next 7 to 10 days, cleansing it after 10 days and repeating the ritual as needed.

MENOPAUSE RITUAL

BEST TIME OF DAY: Anytime
TIME NEEDED: 20 minutes
FREQUENCY: As frequently as needed
ITEMS NEEDED: Garnet, K2, lapis lazuli, sea salt, and a water basin

Menopause signifies a time in a woman's life when she is no longer allocating energy toward reproduction or child rearing. This allows your feminine energy to be woven into other spaces, mainly for yourself and your connection to the Universe. It is called the dark of the moon, similar to the new moon energy, as you are in the space of the void, in direct relationship with the cosmos. You have so much life experience and knowledge, and this time is about sharing that wisdom and medicinal magic with your community and deepening your connection to beyond. This ritual opens the pineal gland and allows for deeper clarity, insight, and wisdom to integrate. These stones also help to cool any sensitivity to heat or hormonal changes underway.

1 Fill the basin with water, and pour in sea salt. Place the garnet in the basin.

2 Hold the lapis lazuli in your right hand and the K2 in your left hand.

3 Sit in a chair and place your feet in the water tub.

4 Let any stress or anxieties release out of your feet into the water, and feel yourself become grounded by the salt water.

5 Begin to call back your energy from the day, week, month, year, or perhaps many years! Set the intention for your own soul energy to return to you, cleansed and clear to integrate back within. Visualize the soul energy as golden threads of light flowing in and weaving back into your energy field.

6 Place your hands on your womb and breathe into your

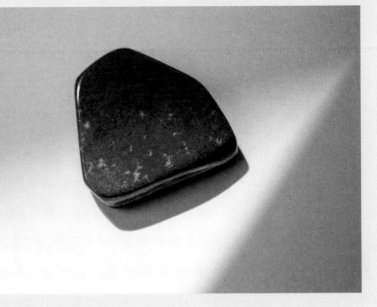

womb (if you no longer have a uterus, the area of your womb).

7   Bring both hands on your heart and breathe into your heart.

8   Bring your right hand (with the lapis lazuli) to your Third-Eye Chakra and your left hand (with the K2) to your womb. Breathe into the ancient wisdom in these stones from ancient civilizations and the ancient wisdom held within your soul. Imagine a line drawn from your Third-Eye Chakra to your womb.

9   Remain here in meditation for a few minutes. Take a deep breath and gently open your eyes. Remove your feet from the water and dry off.

10 Repeat as often as needed with cold water for hot flashes and mood swings.

NEW MOON RITUAL

BEST TIME OF DAY: During the new moon
TIME NEEDED: 15 to 30 minutes
FREQUENCY: Once a month, within 48 hours of the new moon
WHAT YOU'LL NEED: Citrine, clear quartz,
moonstone, and selenite or juniper.

The new moon is the dark of the moon, a place of rebirth and of deep openings for expansion. It is a fertile time for planting seeds, both literally and figuratively, and allowing them to gain strength and power with the growing light of the moon. The new moon is the space of the void, from which all of creation can be born. It is a great time to set intentions, launch projects, work with dreams, and allow time for creative practices. Allow this ritual to tune you into what you want to create and embody throughout the next moon cycle.

1 Energetically cleanse yourself with juniper or a selenite wand.

2 Close your eyes and allow your breath to deepen and expand.

3 Find a seated position, and place the citrine, clear quartz, and moonstone in front of you.

4 Envision the expansive sky overhead. It's a dark inky sky, void of moonlight, full of bright stars and of fertile potential. Tune into your heart and what it is you wish to create in the next new moon cycle.

5   Ask yourself:

    What do I want to create? How can I serve others? How might I practice more self-love? What do I wish to experience? Where can I find more flow? What am I grateful for?

6   Consider your responses to these questions, and choose a word for this moon cycle.

7   Write your word and intentions for this new moon cycle on a piece of paper. You might decorate or color this page with images or colors that inspire you for the month.

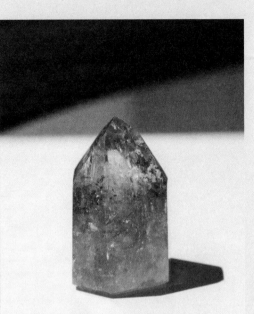

8   Place the citrine, clear quartz, and moonstone vertically along your sheet of paper, and place it on your altar or somewhere you can see it. Reaffirm your intentions every day for the next 30 days.

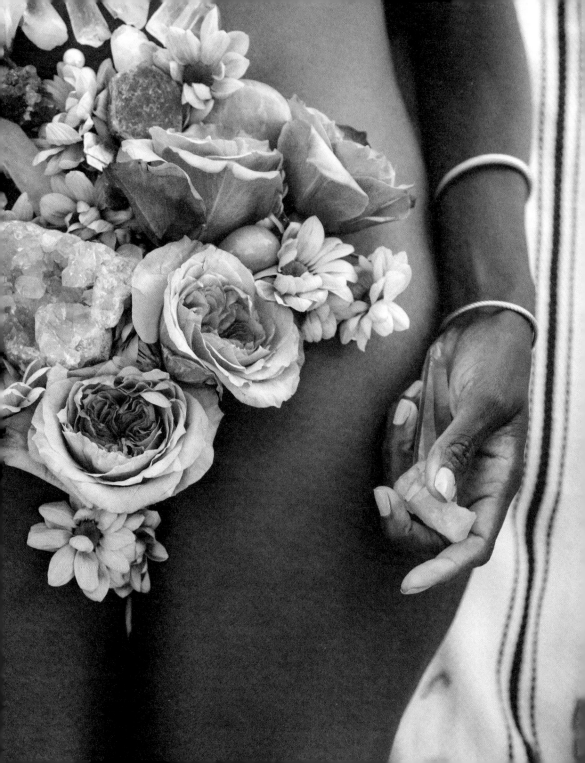

AWAKENING THE DIVINE FEMININE RITUAL

BEST TIME OF DAY: Anytime
TIME NEEDED: 15 to 30 minutes
FREQUENCY: As frequently as needed
WHAT YOU'LL NEED: Kunzite, Lemurian seed,
moonstone, pearl, ruby, and flower petals of any
kind; rose or lavender essential oil (optional)

The Divine Feminine energy is awakening within us collectively and rising to help restore balance and harmony on Earth. While we all have both masculine and feminine energy within, the Divine Feminine is the energy of Mother, the Maiden, the Enchantress, the Crone. It is the energy of Earth herself and of the goddess, the mother and creator of all. We need this energy to awaken so that we might come back into harmony with nature and one another. Use this ritual as needed to connect to the radiant Divine Feminine within you. The ritual may be done in a ritual bath or lying down. If in a bath, add flower petals and rose or lavender essential oil. If you feel called, you may also create a Divine Feminine altar with flowers, photos, prayers, and crystals from the ritual to activate this energy.

1 Lie down on your back. Place the ruby on your pubic bone, the moonstone on your womb, the pearl on the center of your chest, and the Lemurian seed on your heart by your collarbone.

2 Close your eyes, let your breath deepen, and bring yourself into your heart.

3 Let yourself travel deeper and deeper into your heart, and visualize yourself surrounded by trees, deep in nature.

continued…

4   You see the colors around you are extremely vibrant, and there is an effervescent sparkle to the clean air. There is a beautiful stream in front of you leading to a sparkling pool of water, where a beautiful glowing female figure appears. She gently motions you toward her. When you get closer, you see she's a radiant goddess, full of grace, strength, and wisdom, and she emanates rays of unconditional love. She carries a vessel in her hands and invites you into the water with her.

5   You notice as you step into the water, you feel light begin to enter all your cells. She gently anoints you with a golden liquid from her vessel, pouring the elixir on your Crown, Third Eye, Heart, and womb. You feel at home and at ease, wrapped in love, and a deep remembrance and knowing arises within.

6   You notice that as she anoints you, the liquid runs down your face and continues to bless your entire body. Your cells feel lighter, more alive, and more vibrant. She looks deep into your eyes, and you realize now that the goddess staring back at you *is* you, and you have once again awakened to the truth of who you are: the Divine Feminine.

7   Remain here for a few moments while soaking up the radiance of your sovereignty.

8   Deepen your breath and come back to the present moment. Feel your breath within your body and your feet on the ground. Gently open your eyes.

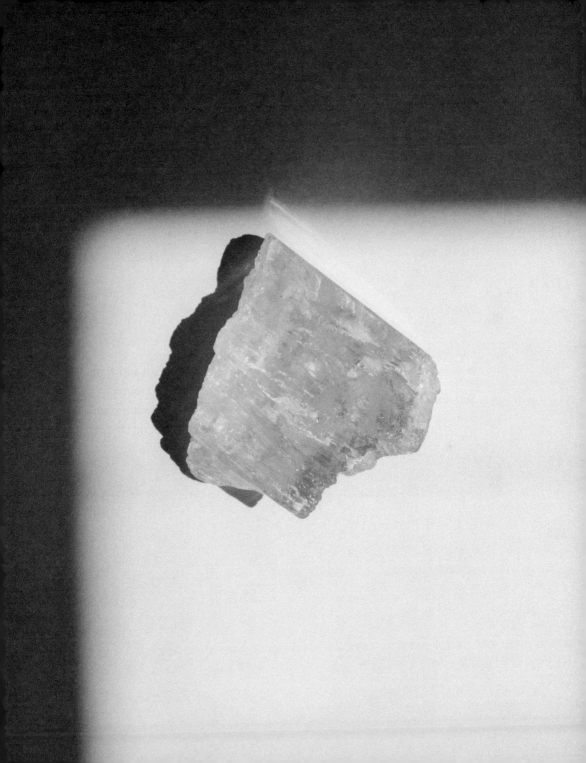

TWELVE

Aligning with the Seasons

WOMEN'S BODIES ARE NATURALLY ALIGNED WITH THE cosmic cycles of the planets. We bleed with the rhythm of the moon cycle, and the four trimesters of pregnancy (the fourth being postpartum) reflect the seasons of the year. The rituals in this chapter help to align your energy and creative force with the seasons of Earth and the cosmos, harnessing the natural energetic portals of those time periods for heightened activation of your intentions.

WINTER SOLSTICE RITUAL

BEST TIME OF DAY: During winter solstice
TIME NEEDED: 15 to 30 minutes
FREQUENCY: Annual
WHAT YOU'LL NEED: Herkimer diamond, sage leaf, and candle

The winter solstice heralds as the darkest day of the year, the celebration of rebirth and the return of the light. This moment of the year is a time for dreaming up new potentials and possibilities for the year to come. It is a time to slow down, get quiet, look within, and acknowledge what was learned and integrated over the last year. Perform this ritual to nourish your mind, body, and spirit to have the energy and stamina come springtime.

1   Find an area where you can create a darkened room. Energetically cleanse yourself with sage and sit down.

2   With your candle in front of you, hold the Herkimer diamond in your hand.

3   Light the candle, then say out loud:

    "I welcome back the light.

    I am grateful for all that has come to pass.

    I honor all that I have done, given, and learned.

    I am grateful for the opportunities to grow and the blessings given.

    I honor the woman I was.

    I honor the woman I am.

    And I honor the woman I will be.

    I welcome back the light."

4   Rest in meditation with the Herkimer diamond. Allow the energy to settle and integrate. You might feel a surge of power or sink into a space of deep peace. Remain here until the energy shifts again and you feel complete.

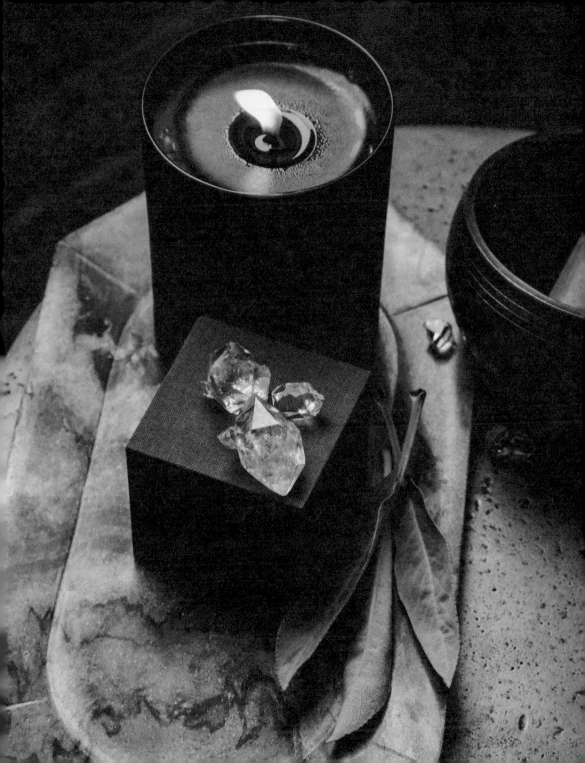

SPRING EQUINOX RITUAL

BEST TIME OF DAY: Midday
TIME NEEDED: 15 minutes
FREQUENCY: Annual, for 3 consecutive days over the spring equinox
WHAT YOU'LL NEED: Black tourmaline, clear
quartz, sunstone, and sage leaf

The spring equinox marks the moment of equal lightness and dark, halfway between the portals of winter solstice and summer solstice. It is a very fertile time of planting literal and figurative seeds for our future. This is a time when the visions from hibernation and dreaming in the winter are planted and begin to take root, a time for honoring new growth and the potential of new life. Perform this ritual the day before, the day of, and the day after the equinox.

Day Before the Equinox

1   Cleanse yourself with sage.

2   Find a comfortable seated position, and hold the black tourmaline in your hand.

3   Set the intention to gently release any fears from the past or old ways of being that are not in alignment with the new you. You might feel a weight in your hands as this energy releases into the black tourmaline, and then a lightness sweeps over.

4   Thank the black tourmaline for transmuting and transforming the energy.

5   Cleanse the stone in a cup of Epsom salts overnight, and throw the salt away in the morning.

Day of the Equinox

1   Try to perform this ritual at the exact time of the solstice, but if that's not possible, anytime within the day is fine.

2   Close your eyes and sit in meditation. Hold the sunstone in your lap with both hands. Feel and visualize the sun pouring through the sky and beginning to charge, cleanse, and neutralize your whole body and energy field.

3   Sense a harmonizing feeling within, a dance of equal balance of dark and light, sun and moon, masculine and feminine. You are both at all times and can hold both in equal harmony.

4   If you already have clarity on the intention you wish to plant into the cosmic ethers, state it out loud now. If you are still discovering this new self, ask for a word or intention to come forth; then remain patient and open to what shows up.

5   Take a few deep breaths, and when you are ready, gently open your eyes.

Day after the Equinox

1   As light is beginning to shine more, it is a great time to set an intention for the next 3 months. Set the intention of the word you received in meditation the previous day. For example, your word could be *grace* or *allow* or *power*.

2   Close your eyes and sit in meditation. Hold your clear quartz. State your intention or word aloud and "into" the crystal. Imagine and feel the vibration of your word(s) being imprinted within the clear quartz.

3   Take a few deep breaths, and when you are ready, gently open your eyes.

4   You may wish to hold your clear quartz every day as a physical reminder of, and to energetically radiate, your intention. You may also place your crystal on an altar or somewhere in your home where you can see it on a daily basis.

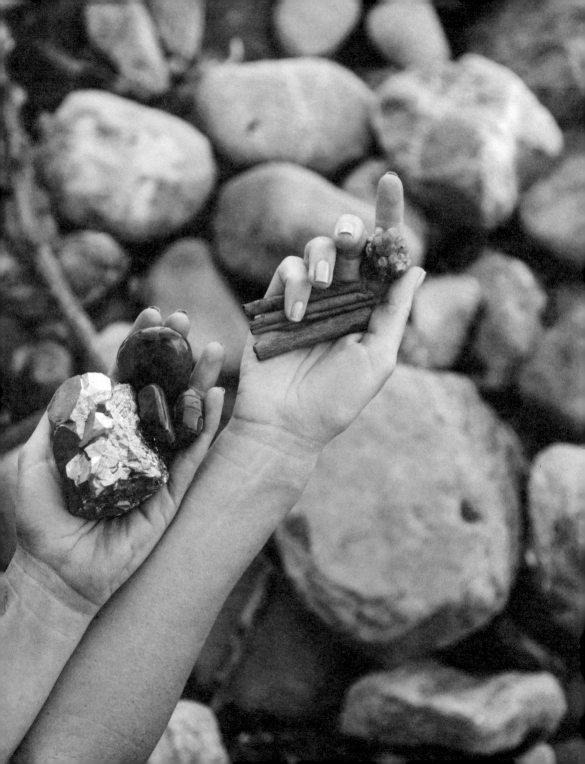

SUMMER SOLSTICE RITUAL

BEST TIME OF DAY: During summer solstice
TIME NEEDED: 20 to 30 minutes
FREQUENCY: Annual
WHAT YOU'LL NEED: Amber, aragonite, carnelian, pyrite,
tiger's eye, cinnamon stick, candle, paper, and pen

Summer solstice marks the longest and brightest day of the year and a day celebrated in many ancient traditions. The powerful, energetically charged summer solstice signifies our fullest potential, personal divine power, and fire within. On this day of new beginnings, what no longer resonates or serves your higher purpose shall be "burned" away. Embrace the radiant light you are, and activate your determination, will, and power within to step into a new expression of yourself. The summer solstice is a great day to be grateful for all the abundance and blessings in life and all that you have learned from your experiences and brought you to this moment right now.

1   Use a cinnamon stick to energetically cleanse yourself.

2   Find a place outside where you can feel the sun on your skin. If it is cloudy or you are unable to get outside, this can all be visualized and performed indoors.

3   Stand with your feet hip distance apart. Place the carnelian directly between your feet, the pyrite in front of you, the tiger's eye to your right, the aragonite directly behind you, and the amber to your left.

continued…

233

4 Raise your hands above your head toward the sun. Feel the warmth on your skin and feel and visualize the prana (life-force energy) and the sun's energy activating your cells.

5 Draw the energy down from the sun with your hands, and bring it to your belly. Feel the divine fire within your incredibly bright self.

6 Repeat this action three times. Draw the energy from the sun to your heart and to your belly. Bring your hands down by your side, palms facing out, and angle your face toward the sun with your eyes closed.

7 Say the following mantra out loud, feeling your power activated as you stand radiant.

"I stand in my true power.

I know who I am.

I give myself permission to fully shine.

I am full of natural abundance and radiance.

I align with my highest self for my highest potential.

I am! I am! I am!"

8 Take a moment and let the energy settle within your body. Feel the natural rush of solar energy and pure power within your being.

9 Take a deep breath in, feel your feet in the earth. Gently open your eyes.

10 You are now walking forth aligned with your highest self and highest possible potential.

FALL EQUINOX RITUAL

BEST TIME OF DAY: During fall equinox
TIME NEEDED: 30 to 45 minutes
FREQUENCY: Annual
WHAT YOU'LL NEED: Garnet, hematite, howlite, candle, pen, and paper

The fall equinox is often referred to as "mid-harvest," when we harvest and reap what we sowed in the spring and worked on in the summer. We can enjoy the fruits of our labor, so to speak. The fall equinox is the balance, the midway point from summer solstice to winter solstice. With the sun shining directly on the equator, it is a day of equal dark and light. As the days grow shorter, we have the opportunity to reassess, regroup, and reorganize, to find balance and take action to get back into alignment. Just as the leaves fall and release, we too can release what no longer serves us in this new chapter.

1 Light your candle and come to a seated position.

2 Place the garnet in your lap, the hematite in your left hand, and the howlite in your right hand.

3 Close your eyes and rest both hands on your knees.

4 Deepen your breath. Bring your energy into your Root Chakra, and feel yourself fully grounded and rooted.

5 Bring your awareness to your Third-Eye Chakra in the center of your forehead and now to your Crown Chakra at the top of your head, allowing them to tingle from your conscious awareness and gently open up.

continued...

235

6   In this open space, ask your highest self:

"Where am I out of balance in my life?

How might I come back into balance?

What action is needed?

Is there a thought pattern or habit that is not supportive and needs to be released?

What is a supportive and nourishing thought or habit that can replace it?"

7   Take a deep breath in and gently open your eyes. Write your insights down in your journal, all except for the negative thought pattern or habit.

8   Write down the old thought pattern or habit on a separate piece of paper. You may choose to consciously burn this paper if you can do so safely in a fireplace or outdoor fire pit, bury it in the ground, or shred it. Allow it to be transmuted in a physical way.

9   Write the new thought pattern or habit on another piece of paper, and stick it somewhere you can see it every day for the next 30 to 60 days, such as in your car, on your phone, or on your mirror.

COSMIC SUPPORT RITUAL

BEST TIME OF DAY: Anytime
TIME NEEDED: 15 to 20 minutes
FREQUENCY: Weekly, daily, or as frequently as needed
WHAT YOU'LL NEED: Apophyllite, azurite,
moldavite, and sage leaf or selenite wand

This ritual brings you back to your innate connection with the cosmos. After all, you are made of literal stardust! The combination of moldavite, azurite, and apophyllite in this Cosmic Support Ritual creates an other-worldly opportunity for expanded awareness and cosmic insight.

1 Energetically cleanse yourself with sage or a selenite wand.

2 Lie down in a comfortable place. Set the moldavite on your heart center, the azurite on your Third-Eye Chakra, and the apophyllite above your head.

3 Close your eyes and deepen your breath. Open your mouth to an O shape, and deeply inhale and exhale through your mouth. Count up 1-2-3 on your inhale and count down 3-2-1 on your exhale. Repeat for 40 to 50 cycles of breath, or about 3 to 5 minutes.

4 Now begin to breathe normally through your nose, allowing your breath to settle into a comfortable pace.

5 Feel the sensations within your body as it is flooded with life force. Feel your connection to all, your cosmic link with all that is. Tune into your awakened Third Eye. Allow whatever visions, memories, images, or geometric shapes to come forth. Let yourself move into a space of expanded conscious awareness! You are the Universe! You are of the stars!

6 Rest here for as long as you wish. When you feel ready, gently open your eyes.

Aligning with the Seasons

REFERENCES

Gagliano, M. "In a Green Frame of Mind: Perspectives on the Behavioural Ecology and Cognitive Nature of Plants." *AoB PLANTS* 7 (2015). doi.org/10.1093/aobpla/plu075.

Gagliano, M. "The Mind of Plants: Thinking the Unthinkable." *Communicative & Integrative Biology* 10, no. 2 (2017). doi.org/10.1080/19 420889.2017.1288333.

Hammerschlag, R., M. Levin, R. McCraty, N. Bat, J. A. Ives, S. K. Lutgendorf, and J. L. Oschman. 2015. "Biofield Physiology: A Framework for an Emerging Discipline." *Global Advances in Health and Medicine* 4, suppl (2015): 35–41. doi.org/10.7453/gahmj.2015.015.suppl.

McCraty, R. (2016). *Science of the Heart, Volume 2: Exploring the Role of the Heart in Human Performance*. An Overview of Research Conducted by the HeartMath Institute. 10.13140/RG.2.1.3873.5128.

McCraty, R., M. Atkinson, and R. T. Bradley. "Electrophysiological Evidence of Intuition: Part 1. The Surprising Role of the Heart." *Journal of Alternative and Complementary Medicine* 10, no. 1 (2004):133–43.

Nautiyal, C. S., P. S. Chauhan, and Y. L. Nene. "Medicinal Smoke Reduces Airborne Bacteria." *Journal of Ethnopharmacology* 114, no. 3 (2007): 446–51. doi.org/10.1016/j.jep.2007.08.038

University of Alabama at Birmingham. "Breakthrough Study Shows How Plants Sense the World: This Understanding Could Help Commercial Crops Resist Pathogens and Drought." ScienceDaily. January 19, 2018. https://www.sciencedaily.com/releases/2018/01/180119190358.htm

Virk, G., G. Reeves, N. E. Rosenthal, L. Sher, and T. T. Postolache. "Short Exposure to Light Treatment Improves Depression Scores in Patients with Seasonal Affective Disorder: A Brief Report." *International Journal on Disability and Human Development* 8, no. 3 (2009): 283–86. doi.org/10.1901/jaba.2009.8-283.

RESOURCES

Crystals and Gemstones

Angelic Healing Crystals
angelichealingcrystals.com

Astara
astaracollective.com

Energy Muse
energymuse.com

Inner Vision Crystals
innervisioncrystals.net

Madagascar Minerals
madagascarminerals.com

Herbs, Resins, and Hydrosols

Anima Mundi Apothecary
animamundiherbals.com

Bulk Apothecary
bulkapothecary.com

Eden Botanicals
edenbotanicals.com

Incausa
incausa.co

Mountain Rose Herbs
mountainroseherbs.com

Pacific Botanicals
pacificbotanicals.com

Essential Oils and Carrier Oils

Floracopeia
floracopeia.com

Living Libations
livinglibations.com

Crystal Singing Bowls

Crystal Tones
crystalsingingbowls.com

Sound Tools

Acutonics
acutonics.com

Sines
sinesmusic.com

Tools for Wellness
toolsforwellness.com

INDEX

ACKNOWLEDGMENTS

To my partner and best friend, Ben, thank you for your unending support, love, and keeping me laughing at all times.

To my mother, thank you for your compassion and dedication to the women of the world.

To my father, thank you for showing me deep reverence of nature, your forever playground.

To Brendan, Vanessa, Solomon, and Stella, thank you for your support and love.

To my incredible friends and soul family, you know who you are, thank you. Your sisterhood and friendship are the sweetest nectar to my soul.

To Meg Ilasco and the wonderful team at Penguin Random House, thank you for believing in me to write this book and for guiding the process. I am forever grateful.

To Amy Dickerson, thank you for bringing this book alive with your magic and beautiful imagery.

To my agent, Brandi Bowles, thank you for your support, encouragement, and continued guidance.

To my many teachers and healers along my path in the seen and unseen, you have all woven your wisdom into my very being and have helped me awaken back home within. I would not be here without your grace and support. Thank you, I deeply and humbly bow. To Jeremy Kennedy, dear friend and cosmic ally, thank you for lending so many of the beautiful stones in this book and sharing your joy and gifts with the world.

To the Divine Feminine in your many forms, thank you for your medicine, magic, guidance, grace, and ever-present truth. To the crystals and the mineral queendom, I am forever in awe, service, and gratitude. Thank you.

ABOUT THE AUTHOR

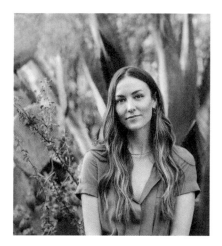

Mariah K. Lyons is a crystal healer, Reiki master, meditation guide, and Western herbalist. She is the founder of ASTARA, a luxury crystalline grounding footwear company integrating ancient healing practices with sustainable design. Her work bridges the world of spirit and matter, and she is deeply dedicated to supporting the awakening of higher consciousness upon the planet through various mediums and healing modalities. Mariah has led workshops and classes for Nike, Yahoo!, NBC Universal, and Dreamworks, and her work has been featured in *Vogue*, the *LA Times*, goop, *Vanity Fair*, *Harper's Bazaar*, and on Good Morning America. She currently resides in Los Angeles, California, with her husband, Ben.

📷

@mariahklyons
@astara